Everything you need to know to help you beat cancer

By Chris Woollams MA (Oxon)

Third Edition: March 2005

Published by:
Health Issues Ltd
The Elms, Radclive Road, Gawcott, Buckingham, MK18 4JB.
Tel: 01280 815166
Fax: 01280 824655
Email: enquiries@iconmag.co.uk

First published June 2002
Second Edition published February 2003
Third Edition published March 2005

Cover design by Jeremy Baker.

ISBN 0-9542968-5-0

Printed in England by Bath Press Ltd, Lower Bristol Road, Bath, BA2 3BL

Dearest Catherine

'It is under the greatest adversity that there exists the greatest potential for doing good, both for oneself and others.'

Tenzin Gyatso,
His Holiness the fourteenth Dalai Lama

Important Notice

This book represents a précis of a vast number of varied sources available to anyone on the subject of cancer, its prevention and cure.

Whilst the author has made every effort to ensure that the facts, information and conclusions are accurate and as up to date as possible at the time of publication, the author and publisher assume no responsibility for errors, omissions, or their consequences.

The author is neither a fully qualified health practitioner nor a doctor of medicine, and so is not qualified to give any advice on any medical matters. Cancer (and its related illnesses) is a very serious and very individual disease. Readers must consult with experts and specialists in the appropriate medical field before taking, or refraining from taking, any action.

This book, and the advice contained, is not intended as an alternative to such specialist advice, which should be sought for accurate diagnosis and before any course of treatment.

The author and the publisher cannot be held responsible for any actions that are taken by any reader as a result of information contained in the text of this book. Such action is taken entirely at the reader's own risk.

Author's Note

This book is the third edition of *Everything you need to know to help you beat cancer*. The first run sold out in less than five months, making it probably the fastest selling cancer book in the UK of all time. All the more remarkable, when you realise that the impetus was generated almost entirely through word of mouth. The phone calls, letters and e-mails have been wonderful. *'Positive'*, *'informative'*, *'easy to read and understand'*, *'inspirational'*, *'down to earth'*, *'practical'*; a phenomenal response from people living with cancer, those who want to prevent it, doctors, nurses, carers, indeed everybody. Thank you.

This third edition has almost 500 new paragraphs containing up-to-date information on cancer prevention and 'cure' including a new section on specific cancers and one on 'the coming cancer cures'. It is our intention to revise the book every year, so that *Everything You Need to Know to Help You Beat Cancer* is always the single fount of knowledge it was intended to be, and truly becomes a 'bible' for anyone wishing to prevent or attempt to beat cancer.

The magazine *Integrated Cancer and Oncology News* (**icon**), is also thriving. It brings up-to-the-minute information, articles and stories to people touched by cancer, doctors, nurses, carers and those who simply want to prevent it. We distribute it free to hospitals, oncology units, support groups, etc, but you can also obtain it by post by simply making a donation to our charity – CANCERactive (see www.canceractive.com).

What started with a book has become a mission. The website www.iconmag.co.uk should be the first port of call for anyone interested in cancer. It has over 700 pages covering all the cancers and all the treatments from surgery to supplements and from chemotherapy to oxygen therapy or photodynamic therapy. We aim merely to keep you informed – you have to make the decisions.

We now have several books: *The Tree of Life: The Anti-Cancer Diet* (a review of which foods, science shows, should be added back into your diet to help beat cancer), *Oestrogen: The Killer in Our Midst* (a look at how this well-known female hormone is linked to all manner of cancers from prostate to breast cancer), *Cancer: Your First 15 Steps* (a simple checklist of what action to take to help your odds of beating cancer – we are aiming to have this given out by doctors at the moment of diagnosis), and finally, out in early 2005, *Conventional Cancer 'Cures' – What's the Alternative?* This book is a patchwork quilt of a number of articles covering developing and clever cancer treatments from around the world.

Finally we are working hard to launch an integrated cancer information centre in the UK and a major offensive on cancer prevention through CANCERactive.

When it all happens we will let you know on our website – this also lists my (now international) speaking venues.

And to think I was happily retired!

CONTENTS

VI.   You really can beat cancer – a summary

FOREWORD

By Dr Diane Keith – a practising general practitioner

There have been many, too many, times in the last 20 years when I have sat in my surgery preparing to tell a patient that they have cancer. It's a disease which occurs with increasing frequency and must be considered of epidemic proportions.

I have to steel myself against the patient's inevitable reaction, when they realise that now, more than ever, they will need a great deal of support.

Obviously my job is to help provide some of that support in whatever way I can, to explain treatments and options, to discuss them all thoroughly, and always, always to give hope.

This is where this excellent book will help patients, their families and doctors alike. It is a mass of widely researched information and jammed full of helpful tips. Frankly, it was a real eye-opener to read just how much is known about cancer and the ways of overcoming it.

Crucially, it can also help non-sufferers; people who are currently healthy and do not want to become merely part of the growing statistics.

This book sets out to provide a simple summary of all the basic information and knowledge you require at your fingertips. It is deliberately written in plain English. And that is just what we all need.

The old expression, never give up, is so true when it comes to the lot of the cancer sufferer, their family, and friends. And this book makes you realise just how much is actually known and available, to make us all feel more optimistic.

It also clarifies one important point: that cancer need not be inevitable, bad luck, or something that runs in the family. With a little effort and sensible self-discipline it can very likely be prevented in the first place.

This book is extensive in its coverage and does not pretend to go into vast detail nor baffle with science. Re-read a chapter again and, if you are not sure about something, go and talk to your GP. Take the book with you.

I commend this book as a valuable extra weapon to all those who want to beat cancer.

I now have something very positive to put into my patients' hands, and I for one, am thankful.

Dr Diane Keith, Surrey, England
June 2002

PREFACE

Over the next few days as you read this book at your leisure, you will come to realise just how much is actually known about cancer; its causes and prevention, its origins and its possible cures.

Depending upon our age, diet and lifestyle, our bodies make between 200 and 1,000 cancer or pre-cancerous cells every day. The statistics show that a cancer will affect one in three of us, and one in four of those affected will die.

But look at these figures another way. Despite producing cancer cells day in, day out, two thirds of us will never contract the disease and, of those who do, 75 per cent will beat it!

Why? Because each of us is a wonderfully tuned and self-protecting living organism, improved and perfected over millions of years to survive most of the harmful things the universe throws our way.

That protection is provided by our **immune system,** the two most important words you need to know when it comes to this subject. You should learn to love your immune system, to nurture it, and maximise it, because you need it in tip-top condition every minute, of every hour, of every day you live. And there are many, many things you can do to strengthen it, just as there are all too many things that you do already that weaken it.

Whilst I do have a strong conviction that cancer is beatable, you need to accept that it occurs through a complex multi-stage process. Beating it is equally a multi-stage task – as individual as each of us is individual. Furthermore, there is no one disease called cancer, any more than there is one form of influenza or one type of cold. Cancer is a generic term for a similar but very individual group of diseases. So this book makes no claims, and offers no promises.

What is clear, is that being healthy cannot be simply regarded as ensuring all your mechanical parts are in working order. Your health stems from your attitude to life, your body's energy systems, endocrine, blood, and lymph systems, well ahead of any problem in a localised area such as your breast or prostate. So when you read the sections on diet, exercise, and supplements understand this: Whilst these areas are crucial to your health, so is your overall happiness, your sense of purpose, the laughter you share with friends and even your sex life. All these things can and do affect your immune system.

A healthy life is about balance. Think of it as a health 'bank balance'. There are constant and increasing drains on your resources, large debits every time you drink too much, smoke or become stressed. But you can cut some of those bills if you want to. You can also do a lot to increase the credit side of your health bank balance as you will see in the sections that follow.

The first aim of this book is to save you time and effort, and to provide you with a complete summary of the basics that I have learned whilst trying to help my daughter with her cancer. I've scoured books and research papers, informed articles and the internet, talked to oncologists (cancer specialists), doctors and alternative health experts.

The second aim was to write a simple book that could not only be read in just a few days, but with a format that would make it a simple reference guide to be returned to, depending upon your specific needs. Whilst the book has breadth, it certainly is not a text book, nor did I want to go too deeply into often complex detail. Of course there is more to find out, more to learn. And because things are changing all the time, I've included a further reading list, helpful phone numbers and internet sites should you want to find out more. **Icon** (Integrated Cancer and Oncology News) magazine will help you in this as will our web site (www.iconmag.co.uk). People often ask me why I haven't included detailed references. Well, firstly because this is supposed to be an easy, non-frightening read for people who have no knowledge of science, clinical trials or medical texts. And secondly, virtually everything is backed up on our website if you do want more information and detail.

This book is a précis of the vast amount of information already in the public domain. Where possible I have tried to highlight both sides of an argument.

I am a biochemist and deal in facts about what affects the cell, its systems, or indeed the whole body. I am not interested in the petty squabbles between individuals in the medical profession and individuals in alternative medicine. Cancer is a serious subject and solutions must be all-embracing, covering everything from surgery to supplements and from radiotherapy to reiki.

Eliminating the cancer tumour rather than the root cause, runs the risk of it returning in the longer term. What is the benefit of chopping out the cancer tumour, if the patient persists with some behaviour that actually caused the original problem, like smoking? True, you buy time with which to analyse the possible causes and ideally correct the underlying problem. But do the patients and the medical profession use that time searching out the causes, the toxins and the lifestyle factors?

Sadly, a lack of time forces too many doctors to focus on the localised cancer and not the whole patient. Yet without any shadow of doubt, cancer is systemic. Its effects can be shown throughout the body even though all you see is a localised bump. Logic dictates then, that for successful 'cure' you need to treat the patient, the whole patient and not merely the lump in her head, breast or arm. The logical aim must be to treat the cause not the symptoms. Yet modern medicine is ever more myopic. Could this be why we see only three out of several hundred cancers where there are full medical cures and why doctors, instead, talk about remission or extending the active life of sufferers? Certainly no one should blame the doctors; they are paid to be experts in surgery, or radiotherapy or chemotherapy. And that's exactly what they are. Indeed they could qualify as doctors without spending a single day learning about nutrition, biochemistry or body energy.

Having explored the topic pretty comprehensively, my conclusion is simple. Most cancers are beatable. There is simply no need to be a statistic in this epidemic if you know what to do, and then take action.

What is clear to me is that we all have to re-educate ourselves. We need to realise that across a vast expanse of time we developed an interdependent and symbiotic relationship with our environment. After millions of years of slow and even negligible change, the last 150 years have produced dramatic changes in our environment and dangers for all of us. Make no mistake about this. Cancer is a modern disease. A study of over 3000 human skeletons in Croatia, spanning 7300 years showed no traces of cancer until the middle of the nineteenth century (*National Geographic*, July 2004). As individuals, we all need to learn the science of cancer prevention; to recreate for ourselves a life from a healthier age.

Every government works on the straight-line principle; namely that next year will be better than this, and the year after better than the last. Recessions are but mere blips in a continuous upward trend. Any biologist will tell you that life just is not like that. All life is cyclical. As populations of animals increase, for example lemmings, they become out of balance with their environment and this in turn provides a restricting and self-limiting control on the population. We might worry about specific problems like nuclear power and possible mishaps, but we give little thought to a lifestyle that involves extensive use of, say, cars and computers, farmed food, and chemical toxins. A sedentary lifestyle, for example, coupled with increasing consumption of fats from farmed animals and fish will ultimately weaken our immune systems. Coupled with other environmentally negative influences, it is highly likely this will 'self regulate' our population. We may be talking decades rather than years, but what will the educated populations think when life expectancy rates start to fall, or when cancer rates double or triple?

Meanwhile such governments aided by the drug companies and charities spend truly vast sums of money on cancer 'cures'. In the year 2000 in the USA those combined forces spent $11bn. Compared to this, the amount spent on cancer prevention was negligible, less than 1 per cent; and even that includes 'screening' which is hardly real prevention. Phrases like, 'locking the stable door after the horse has bolted', spring to mind.

Recent Cancer Research UK figures show an annual growth of individual cancer cases of roughly 2 per cent. But somehow skin cancer, the fastest growing UK cancer, was omitted from the figures. With this included, cancer cases have grown almost 4 per cent per year for the last 25 years! This, despite an attack on smoking in the UK.

Within this worsening big picture, I believe it is still possible for you to create your own highly successful micro-environment and this book will help you. Getting 'back to basics' is an important start. The basis of cancer prevention is common sense. Try to cut the unnecessary toxins out of your life and add back in the things that will boost your immune system to its maximum. Vote with your feet and your wallet.

The great majority of cancer sufferers are not victims. Few are unlucky and catch it from some passing stranger by, say, viral infection. Prevention is in your own hands. And cure is available for almost everybody who is prepared to be positive, more open-minded and more all embracing of the knowledge and facts that exist.

———————————

Finally I'd like to say a personal thank you to the people who helped with the original book, and those who have helped with this edition, or should I say mission! Dr Diane Keith, Larry Brooks, Richard Waters, Marie Pay and especially to Lindsey Fealey and the team at **icon**. Your comments and help were invaluable.

Chris Woollams
February 2005

INTRODUCTION

Catherine

My daughter Catherine is 26 years old, happy, fun loving, good looking and clever. She has a chemistry and law degree from Bristol University. She also has cancer.

Over the weekend of the 21 April 2001 we were celebrating my second daughter's 18th birthday with a Saturday dinner, and a Sunday lunch, so the headache on Monday morning was not entirely unexpected, although the sickness was. By Tuesday evening St Thomas' Hospital in London had given her a scan and we were told Catherine had a brain tumour.

The health system went into overdrive and I have nothing but praise. Catherine was transferred to Queen Square in London to the National Hospital for Neurology, and we were told she would be operated on the following Saturday. No words can express how rapidly your life can change, how the happiness of a birthday weekend could be followed by the crushing horror, fear and sadness of a life-threatening operation to your 'baby'.

The excellent surgeon, Mr Kitchen, came out of theatre to tell me that 'the operation went without incident'; (no emotional extremist can presumably even apply to be a brain surgeon). And Catherine seemed to heal by the second during the five days that followed. We were told that small brain tumours were not uncommon; that they had taken most but not all out and with Catherine's age and health, there was little to worry about.

The following Friday we were told what remained of the tumour was malignant.

My personal background included four years at Oxford University reading biochemistry, with a year specialising in cancer research and viruses. Although I was asked to stay on for a doctorate in cancer research, I am afraid the call of capitalism

1

was too strong and I spent the next 22 years in advertising and marketing, in the end building a group of nine companies which we put on the stock market. Then I retired aged 45.

Actually I say retired, but it is not a word that really figures in my personal vocabulary. Over the next five or six years I helped some friends launch companies, but my real interest was a personal quest to understand what things really make a person healthy.

So I read and read, primarily about nutrition, but that spun off into an interest in anti-ageing and body energy systems. Just for fun I did a reiki course and even became a personal trainer, and my business experience helped to launch two health clubs for Virgin.

When Catherine was first diagnosed I did what any good father, biochemist and marketing man would do. I did my homework. I rang experts in the USA, the UK, and France, gleaned information and second opinions from medical and alternative experts, read so many books we could have opened our own health library, and became a regular on the internet.

I came to five crucial conclusions:

*Firstly, **there is so much information out there, if you have the time and the inclination to look.** However, few scientists seem to be even telling each other (and as a result there are frequently similar research studies in different areas of the world!), let alone passing it on to GPs and patients. Even the oncologists have trouble keeping up with it all.*

*Secondly, just when you need it, **there is no single source, no fount of knowledge,** no 'cancer bible' you can turn to for an easy read. Something that might save you six month's work. Something that might put together the very best of orthodox and complementary therapies.*

*Thirdly, there is a saying that knowledge is power. With cancer, knowledge is the difference between life and death. But the fact that much of the latest information is not getting through to GP's and even oncologists means that people are not dying of cancer; **people are dying of ignorance.***

Fourthly, you will find that throughout this book I keep repeating the phrase 'there is so much you can do to increase your odds of beating cancer'. From acupuncture to supplements, or exercise and diet. Sadly, the onus for building this 'total package' of activities lies with you and no one else.

Lastly, do everything in your power not to get cancer in the first place. Spending some time and effort adopting a new lifestyle with the help of this book will give you an invaluable insurance policy in terms of prevention. And my main piece of advice is: 'Love your immune system'!

Catherine had lots of questions that deserved and demanded definitive, factual answers. And so we come to this book. I hunted high and low to get answers. The problem for most people is that they simply do not have the time to read hundreds of books, articles and look at internet sites, especially if they are suffering from cancer. Worse, some of the books need a biochemist to understand them, whilst others are too simplistic, and most only cover a part of the information available. Some are very personal and relate to an individual cancer, and all too many deteriorate into a glorified recipe book without the glossy photographs.

The great majority also seem to dwell on the problems and the morbid statistics in their opening chapters. This just puts the cancer sufferer into more despair. As Catherine said to me: "Dad, I'm not interested in cancer. I'm interested in living!"

Catherine was asking questions that went right across the disease from A to Z, and although we did find all the answers we wanted, we simply couldn't find them in one place.

But then came the defining moment: the real raison d'être for my pieces of paper to come together in a 'Cancer Prevention and Cure Bible'.

Catherine and I were with her oncologist discussing her radiotherapy some four weeks into the six week course. He had already informed her that her chances of surviving five years were approximately 15 per cent, so we knew the seriousness of the situation.

I asked him one straightforward question: 'Exactly what supplements would you give Catherine to improve her chances and the radiotherapy's performance?' To which he replied, 'Well you're the biochemist, you'd know better than me!'.

Saying that I wanted to give her a detox, he replied, 'I don't know what you mean by detox – if you mean antioxidants I'm against them because I read in the paper that they give them to astronauts to prevent the negative effect of radiation in space. But I want the radiation to work'. I interjected that, "Vitamin E would not some-how mystically shield a cancer cell but promote the immune system and selenium .....". He cut me off to say that they had conducted tests and shown that selenium supplements improved the effective-ness of radiotherapy, as did soya isoflavones.

All I could say was, 'When did you intend to tell us this?' and vow to myself that I'd write down all my research findings in a single source, in plain simple English, with no complex and baffling scientific or medical jargon, for everybody's benefit. Fortunately, we already had Catherine on selenium and isoflavones, but if I hadn't been a biochemist or done my home-work how would we have known?

Perhaps I'm being a bit naughty here. In my view Catherine would not have survived without surgery, radiotherapy and the excellence of her doctors. And the doctors are trained to think in terms of something called 'best practice', which means that they are encouraged to use a fomulaic approach largely relying on surgery, radiotherapy and chemotherapy and are not encouraged to think 'outside of the box'. Their training leads them to pre-scribe things that have gone through a Government Health Department specified system of testing. Selenium and isoflavones haven't had such proper 'clinical trials' completed and without this formal data, doctors are not in a position to make hard and fast recommendations. If there is a fault, it clearly lies in the system not the people working in it.

With Catherine I became her manager and the 'nag', ringing her up about diet, chasing her with supplements, encouraging her into yoga, sending her to cranial osteopaths, and arranging trips to shows and events to maintain her positive attitude. We even planned to launch a monthly cancer help magazine, which was not only much needed but could give her a sense of purpose.

I am pleased to say this project reached fruition with the launch of **icon** *(Integrated Cancer and Oncology News) in July 2002. It launched with sixteen pages and now, nearly three years*

later is forty-four pages, free in hospitals and written by profes-
sional journalists from information supplied by doctors and
professors from around the world.

It has been a great success, and is a way of keeping people
up-to-date with all the latest news as well as sharing their
ideas and experiences. We have also launched our website
www.iconmag.co.uk which we hope will be the first port of call for
anyone interested in beating cancer. Again it is in the same style: an
'integrated' approach to cancer; informative and inspirational.

If you are unfortunate enough to contract cancer you have to
muster every armament you can to aid your fire-power and rid
yourself of it. You need to go to an oncologist who is experienced
in your type of cancer, who is fighting alongside you and provid-
ing you with lots of useful information. A friend whose daughter
had skin cancer said her specialist gave her computer printouts
and photostats an inch thick so that she could be fully informed.
Don't settle for less. Ask and be pushy because the standards of
support vary so much between specialists. If you are going to
homeopaths, cranial osteopaths or healers, go to experts on your
type of cancer. Get second and third opinions from people with
recent experience, and check and double-check their opinions
and recommendations.

Someone has to manage and co-ordinate the multitude of treat-
ments available. The cancer patients themselves will become
depressed, through circumstance, or treatment or both, and a
friend or relative must take on the role of minder (even though
I'm sure Catherine wished I'd go away on many occasions).

Finally though, I believe beating cancer is about odds and,
*particularly, improving your odds. **If you get cancer you do not***
want to be the average case.

With Catherine we have done everything in our power to
increase the odds in her favour.

Through Western diet, being overweight, smoking, drinking,
and pollution, the odds on you contracting cancer are increasing,
if you just go with the flow.

As Samuel Johnson said, 'The chains of habit are too weak to
be felt until they are too strong to be broken'. With the modern
world dragging you into bad habits, only serious self-discipline

will get you out of becoming more and more at risk.

There is no doubt that at university Catherine had fallen into bad habits. These, coupled with an ongoing illness that was never adequately addressed, worsened her odds to the point where a cancer developed.

We believe we have learned what caused her cancer and what was sustaining it. This aligned with some excellent modern medical care, numerous 'complementary health' treatments and a whole re-education process on her diet and lifestyle, have increased Catherine's odds for survival. Catherine herself has been absolutely brilliant and completely reinvented herself in terms of diet, lifestyle, exercise, and attitude. Above all, her determination and the wonderful support of her friends (and she has many) helped this enormously. But we are realists. As one professor said to me, 'trying to cure a glioblastoma is a bit like trying to swing a tiger by its tail'.

But this book is actually for people who want to prevent the onset of cancer just as much as it is for those with cancer. In both cases increasing the odds is about knowing the facts and understanding likely causes and likely solutions. The self-discipline needed simply needs to be even more rigorous if you have already contracted cancer.

So I pass on my answers to Catherine's questions to anybody who wants to read them. I hate to think that a lack of information, or worse misinformation, would result in any more unnecessary deaths when so much hard evidence is available, if only one knew where to start looking.

No one wants cancer. Now I've seen it first hand I can assure you it is a dreadful problem to have. Everybody should do everything in their power to prevent themselves from getting it.

Hopefully this book is a good place to start.

SECTION I

A guide to cancer in
plain English

Introduction

"I went into a pub and asked for a quickie. I think you'll find that it's pronounced quiche, said the barmaid."

(Italian Ambassador Luigi Amaduzzi on the perils of speaking a foreign language).

That's also the first problem with cancer – with all those technical terms, it's like trying to understand a foreign language. So I'll keep it simple, and non-technical! UK research has shown that cancer patients simply do not understand 'cancer speak' from their doctors.

Q1. What is cancer?

A cancer tumour starts with an initial rogue cell. If it beats your body's defence systems it behaves like a foetal cell dividing and copying itself very rapidly, but in an uncontrolled manner. Since such cells can divide as often as once every 20 minutes, the original rogue cell can grow into a tumour very quickly.

A tumour is an unusual growth in the body. Some tumours are benign (ie grow at only a modest rate and do not spread); whilst some are malignant (ie grow rapidly and do spread within that tissue or to other parts of the body). This malignancy is what is commonly described as cancer.

Cells from the core tumour can break away acting as 'negative disciples', sending out the havoc message to other places in the body (metastasis). When this message reaches another part of the body, it can simply start another tumour there.

A friend of mine was an expert in lasers. His wife had a breast tumour. He actually developed a laser himself to shine on her body that would show up the tumour. In fact he found nine such 'hot spots' all over her body.

The original tumour is called the primary, the new tumours in other parts of the body are called secondaries. Some tumours, for example primary brain tumours, are confined to such tight spaces that they have difficulty sending out rogue messages. More often though, tumours, for example breast tumours, not only send out the rogue message to places like the liver or brain where they can initiate secondaries, but often the rogue messengers collect in the lymph nodes. This is because of the action of the body's immune defence system which has carted off a couple of rogue cells to the lymph nodes in order to study them and try to produce a neutralising antibody. The rogue cancer cells actually collect in and 'poison' the very cells that are trying to eradicate them (this will be explained in far more detail in Section II).

Even in normal healthy people several hundred initial rogue cancer and pre-cancer cells are made every day, but these are rendered harmless through the body's various immune defence systems.

So there are a number of opportunities to control cancer: For example, stopping the initial rogue cells forming, neutralising the rogue cells as effectively as possible; stopping possible tumour growth; preventing the rogue cells from spreading.

Q2. What 'causes' a cancer cell?

The World Health Organisation has said that, of the 6 million worldwide cancer cases each year, about 3 million were caused by poor diet, 1.5 million by infection and 1.5 million by toxins in the environment.

I'm not sure it can be put in boxes like this, especially since they make no acknowledgement of the role of factors such as stress or mental attitude. I believe it is perhaps more relevant to say that poor diet, toxins and infection can all cause a fundamental weakening of our immune systems, making cancer more likely.

A number of degenerative diseases are thought to be caused by a 'triple whammy' and cancer almost certainly arises in the same way.

Firstly, you may have some genetic predisposition or weakness. However, in the case of cancer, this is probably inherent in nearly all of us.

If you take people from China or Japan, where certain cancers hardly exist, and subject them to Western pollution, diet and lifestyle, their rates of cancer increase in line with the native inhabitants indicating that most people are actually predisposed to cancer. However, it has been estimated from research studies that some people actually have genetic 'faults', which causes them to feel that cancer 'runs in the family' and that they have a higher risk. Six or seven per cent of people are affected like this. However, even if this is the case, there is a great deal you can do to avoid it, and your chances of success with the right tactics are high.

Secondly, you need a negative environment in and around the cell.

This can be caused by diet or specifics like tobacco, sunlight, pesticides, and toxins in everyday products; in fact a whole host of things including stress. In one region of Africa the bite of a fly causes the weakness.

Every one of us has an immune system, our natural defence against foreign invaders like viruses. This system will usually recognise a rogue cell or its message and attempt to neutralise it.

13

In a healthy body under normal conditions, rogue cells are mopped up all the time. But, the effects of a poor diet, pesticides, smoking, alcohol, excess fats, and age, weaken the immune system. Sometimes it is stretched to breaking point dealing with the production of rogue cells.

Thirdly, you need 'the final straw', something to tip your biological balance over the edge.

If, for example, on top of everything else the body gets an infection which further weakens the immune system, the rogue cells will start to win their battle. Since the immune system weakens markedly with age, for reasons we will explore later, this 'triple whammy' is most often seen with older people. But not always.

The idea that you probably need all three factors explains why some diseases (e.g. heart problems, high cholesterol) run in families, yet some members can and do avoid them. But they avoid them by not falling into the same traps as their other family members, for example, by watching their diet or taking exercise. Recent research on inherited diseases in Scandinavia using twins supports this totally. The *New England Journal of Medicine* reports on 4,788 pairs of twins from Scandinavia who were studied, and concluded that, 'Inherited genetic factors make a minor contribution to the susceptibility of most types of cancer'. The USA National Cancer Institute said, 'This study should dispel the fatalism of the general public that if it runs in my family, I'm doomed'.

Cancer, like heart disease, can be avoided and beaten if you take positive action and work at it.

It demands effort and discipline in a world that is actively and increasingly working against you. Make no mistake, there are many things you can do to prevent or stop cancer.

The Chinese have a saying, 'Treating a person when they become ill is like starting to dig a well when you are thirsty.'

From the cancer patients I have seen and talked to, I counsel everyone to do everything in their power to avoid getting cancer in the first place. And to cancer sufferers I would say, 'Think very seriously about what diet, lifestyle and psychological problems might have caused the cancer and work hard to undo the damage.' You can do it if you really want to.

Q3. How does a cancer cell develop?

The truth is that scientists are not exactly sure! There are several theories. Indeed there may even be several different types of cancer development processes (see page 235 for one of them). Here I give you the most popular 'orthodox' view!

Every cell in your body has a nucleus, the 'control centre' for your whole body and your whole life. Inside it is your DNA, which I want you to imagine as a very, very long but infinitesimally fine string wrapped up in a tight ball.

Along the length of this DNA string is a code made up of a sequence of chromosomes unique to you. This is your personal blueprint, and it sends out messages telling your body to make five fingers, two legs, blue eyes and blond hair. The ball is loosely 'glued' together by histamines and other substances. Some parts of the ball of string are exposed to the outside world, other parts are not.

Inside the nucleus you also have substances which work like little trains. On the string there are little 'start' points and little 'stop' points.

The trains see a start point, jump on and go along the string until they hit a stop point. They then fall off. The code in between the start and stop is read by the train, which copies it and sends the exact copy off as a message to the world outside the nucleus. Obviously the trains can only read a full sequence if it is exposed and not buried deep inside the ball.

Imagine that one day the effect of your lifestyle, diet, and an infection all cause the ball of string to be surrounded by toxins, which have found their way into the nucleus and the fluid around the ball of string. The toxins may attack the string and even unravel it slightly. Other bits of code are suddenly freed to be read, and other start and stop points are seen by the train. So it reads them and sends out new messages.

Almost all of these messages may be gobbledegook and mean nothing to the systems around the body reading them. The body's immune system simply rejects and neutralises them rendering them harmless. Others though can be rogue cancer cell precursors.

15

In fact you need to imagine our ball as having two parts, a red part and a smaller blue part. The blue part itself actually has an in-built protective part, a gene, a defence system to recognise when the DNA string has gone wrong and is a potential rogue. It can repair damage to our string or order the body to neutralise any rogue messages produced.

Some rogues may get past this blue defence system, but the healthy body has a second line of defence, a strong immune system, which is ready for these 'escapees' and mops them up.

There are a number of ways in which the original messages can be rogue. Sometimes toxins cause chromosomes to stick together, sometimes a bit breaks off. Sometimes bits become reassembled in the wrong order. Rarely, too, the DNA isn't copied perfectly when the original cell divides to make new ones, so an ABCDE code becomes ABXDE.

The point is that whatever the particular detailed explanation of a rogue message, it is invariably formed by the DNA string ball being bathed in toxins inside the nucleus.

These toxins or poisons cause the attack on the ball of string and the malfunctioning and misreading to take place.

All remains manageable as long as the blue defence system in the DNA string works and/or the overall immune system is strong. But what happens when the actual piece of DNA that is your front line defender is the piece that is poisoned, and it is the blue part that sends out a cancer message?

Up to half of all cancers are thought to be caused by the 'defender' portion of the DNA itself going wrong or simply not working. Smoking, UV light, asbestos and many more substances can cause this.

In this case a rogue message breaks out with no 'front line' DNA defence to stop it and, if it beats the more general immune system too, becomes a cancer cell, then a cancer tumour.

These cancer cells are clever. The rogue message can take advantage of a weak immune system but, worse, sometimes it can actually fool the immune system into thinking it is a normal cell. And then the immune system lets it grow!

When a tumour gets to a size of about one centimetre it also needs a blood supply, and it is at this time it starts to grow unchecked. Restricting the growth of the specific blood supply is also an opportunity in our attempt to control cancer.

As you can see, this is a complex multi-step process (in fact far more complex than I have actually described) and it makes it all the more likely that only rarely does only one factor cause the cancer. This is why people with several 'problem factors', for example, poor environment, poor diet, smoking and alcohol, significantly worsen their odds. Again, everyone of us should recognise this fact.

We should also recognise that within our total treatment plan we should include elements that can 'correct' each of the various multi-steps. Some active ingredients of foods can 'correct' the original rogue formation, whilst others are known to tackle metastasis (spread) or the formation of the tumour's blood system. As this book develops you will start to build a positive picture of all the things you can (and need to) do in your cancer-defeating programme!

Q4. How does my DNA become 'poisoned'?

Imagine your cell looking like a poached egg in a pot of water. The yolk is the nucleus, inside which sits your ball of string, the DNA bathed in fluid. In the white of the egg, the cellular liquid, are lots of little power stations called mitochondria, which burn sugar by a process called the Krebs cycle to provide energy for the cell to function. Surrounding the cell, our whole egg, is water or 'lymph'. Beyond the water is the blood system with blood flowing within a more structured tube-like system. Each element of this cellular, lymph and blood system is separated from the next by a membrane largely made up of protein and fats.

Day in, day out, the power stations burn fuel and oxygen to make energy, and waste products are produced. Proteins and fats come into the cell because they are needed to rebuild the cellular structures, like the DNA string itself or the membranes. All these nutrients pass from the blood to the lymph to the cellular liquid (the cytoplasm) and some into the nucleus.

So our ball of string ends up surrounded by a fluid in which there are waste products and inbound nutrients. Worse, some irregular fuels cause the power stations to emit nasty black smoke, which makes the whole environment in there very unpleasant. Some inbound substances also have a polluting effect on our egg yolk.

Also, some of the things coming from the blood system via the lymph may not be nutrients but may themselves be pollutants; for example, the by-products of smoking, or drinking alcohol.

The nastiest pollutants are called free radicals, and their action is to change the molecules they bump into, in the same way that air turns a half-eaten apple brown. This process is called oxidation. They do this because they are incomplete and have a loose, sticky end, which rips parts off other molecules. These damaged molecules in turn can attack others, starting an ongoing chain reaction.

Free radicals are aggressive and they may well attack our DNA string causing it to change structurally. It should be noted that there is some evidence that taking iron supplements actually heightens this aggression and, for example, many anti-ageists steer clear of supplements containing inorganic iron.

The crucial point is that you can make your egg white and egg yolk more polluted by, for example, what you burn at the power stations; or by having stagnant, polluted surrounding lymph preventing the toxins leaving the whole cell. If your blood is carrying high levels of toxins, so too will be your lymph and then your cell. So the DNA string is increasingly surrounded by

- More cell produced toxins
- More 'ingested' toxins.

The body does have a double protection system for mopping up free radicals (as we will see in more detail later) namely

- Antioxidants
- Hormones.

Both of these specifically neutralise free radicals. But, especially as you age, the flow of lymph past the cell is reduced resulting in more waste build-up, and the level of hormones acting to neutralise free radicals decreases.

––––––––––

You may remember from your school days that you can take a beaker of blue liquid, separate it from a beaker of clean water by a membrane or filter paper and, after a reasonable period of time, half the blue will go across into the original jar of clean water. It's called osmosis and happens until the liquid on the two sides of the filter membrane is at the same concentration. Well, that is pretty much how the waste moves out of the egg yolk (the nucleus) into the white (the cell) and into the watery lymph.

In your school experiment, if you wanted more of the blue to go you had to keep changing the beaker of clean water. So too with lymph. It needs to be clean and flowing to take away the maximum amount of waste. If it is not, then the DNA string in our nucleus may, before too long, be swimming in very polluted and toxic fluid.

––––––––––

In summary

- Do not ingest unnecessary extra toxins
- Keep your lymph clean and flowing (e.g. by drinking lots of water and by your own 'movement', which we will explain in Q5)
- Keep your level of antioxidants and hormones up, especially as you age
- Do not over-stress your cellular biochemistry by making the power stations produce excess waste.

With regard to the last point, it is not just the case that burning nasty fuels can over pollute a cell; both an excess of stress hormones or exercising too strenuously will encourage the power stations to work at inefficient levels and produce excess waste.

Cancer cells are different

The poisoning of your cells renders them different in several ways.

One fact is that the power stations, or mitochondria, in a cancer cell are very different from those in normal cells.

Under normal conditions a healthy cell produces its energy in the power stations by burning carbohydrates in oxygen. If the cell has become toxic, the process becomes less efficient, using less oxygen, producing more acidic and toxic by-products and providing less energy. All this causes a vicious circle to occur with the power station becoming less and less efficient and using even less oxygen and powering the whole cell downwards. Cancer cells do not use oxygen, in fact they thrive in its absence and can be killed by its presence, as was shown by Nobel Prize winner, Otto Warburg in 1931.

A major by-product of this oxygen-free process is lactic acid, more commonly known as the cause of cramp in athletes' muscles. The lactic acid can only be neutralised if it can be taken away via the lymph and blood to the liver, an organ already over-worked in a cancer patient. The end product of the neutralising process is glucose, which is also the favourite food of a cancer cell. So you see that cancer cells are clever, and set up their own 'self-feeding' process in your body!

This may all seem a little complicated but it provides further lessons:

- Keep your system 'oxygenated' through exercise, deep breathing, clean air.
- Keep your blood and lymph systems clean and moving.
- Keep your liver healthy.
- Minimise your intake of glucose, the favourite food of cancer cells.

Q5. How can I reduce the effect of toxins?

Even if you ate only organic food, used only non-toxic toiletries, drank only the purest water, never touched red meat or dairy products, never smoked or drank alcohol and lived the purest of lives, you would still build up toxins in your body. A number of eminent cancer experts feel that over time it is inevitable that high levels of toxic wastes build up in and around the cell, and this accounts for the fact that 80 per cent of cancers occur in the over 60 age group.

But it is not inevitable.

Move your lymph

As we have said, toxins inside the cell move into the liquid outside the cell (the lymph) and are taken away. The lymph then passes them into the blood system which takes it via the liver and kidneys to be excreted. So the lymph plays a crucial role in keeping your cells toxin free.

However, unlike the blood system where the action of the heart keeps it moving, the lymph, which has twice the total volume of the blood in your body, has little or nothing to keep it flowing – except for your own activity.

If you are dehydrated or inactive you will build up more toxins around your cells.

Activities like t'ai chi, or aerobic exercise (which encourages the pumping of the blood and in turn massages the lymph system into action) move the toxins out. But this only does part of the job. The most important thing to do every day is to open up your chest by moving your arms wide. This is because the largest channel of lymph, called the thoracic duct, lies across the chest and stimulating movement of this is crucial to good lymph flow.

Swimming is excellent, especially the breaststroke. Press-ups are also good. Certain yoga exercises, like the salutation to the sun, the cobra and the shoulder stand, really get the thoracic lymph moving. Even laughing deeply massages the thoracic duct, as does deep breathing (which is an important aspect of yoga. Interestingly it is also an important part of Chinese cancer therapy.)

Sleep also aids lymph movement, because when you are horizontal it does not have to fight gravity. Conversely, people who don't stand up straight risk restricting their thoracic lymph flow.

Massage, particularly deep massage such as Thai massage or shiatsu, stimulates the lymph system and gets it moving. The term lymphatic drainage is often correctly applied to this form of massage.

Detoxification and fibre

Regular bowel movements and a clean liver also help to detoxify the cellular system. Everybody should ensure they have:

- A good intake of fibre from plants, vegetables and fruits (psyllium seeds are a good addition to breakfast cereals).

A diet high in fibre is directly linked to reduced body toxins and high fibre in the colon helps carry more toxins and, for example, excess hormones out of the body. But it is not just in the bowels that fibre does its work. Phytates and lignans, two commonly occurring substances in plant fibre, stick to the free radicals and neutralise them, like the actions of antioxidants beta-carotene and lycopene. Which is why diet is so important in reducing the toxic waste in and around cells.

- A good intake of water throughout the day, especially after exercise or massage.

This is essential to flush toxins out of the blood and lymph. The accepted view is that you should drink at least 1.5 litres per day but an eminent bottled water company admitted to me that there is no research to support this. It is felt by many medical practitioners that many of us are dehydrated and there is a lot of justification in encouraging all of us to consume at least 1.5 litres per day (but not with meals as it dilutes the enzymes needed for proper food digestion).

- A detox once per month for at least three to four days.

The issue of detoxing produces heated debate in some medical quarters but users feel strongly about the benefits. The whole area of juice diets and detoxing will be covered later in the book.

Boost your natural defences

The biggest neutraliser of the toxins and free radicals is the immune system aided and abetted by the endocrine system.

Research is quite clear that taking beta-carotene, vitamin C and vitamin E, for example, boosts the neutralising ability of the immune system. (Please beware of beta-carotene if you smoke.)

There are foods with antioxidant ingredients like turmeric, garlic and echinacea that will improve the 'quality' of your immune system so it can better recognise the rogue cells.

Hormones such as growth hormone, melatonin and DHEA also significantly help to 'mop up' free radicals as do a number of co-factors like coenzyme Q10 (CoQ10) – all will be covered in more detail in question 18. Unfortunately all the latter four 'good guys' peak in the body between the ages of 16–20 and then steadily decrease to the point of almost non-existence by the age of 70. This is a crucial reason for excess toxic waste in old people.

The good news is you can do something about this. For example, experiments with people over 60 taking 60 mgs per day of CoQ10 for three months returned them to levels found in 20 year olds. We shall see later that you can take action to keep your hormone levels as high as possible as you age.

Having a slightly alkaline body (in a world where most of us have an acid body) is essential to the proper working of the immune system. Stress, smoking, alcohol and a poor diet will all make your cells more acid and your immune system less effective.

Omega 3 has a huge effect on detoxing the cellular surroundings, as does providing a good supply of oxygen.

Acidophilus and other 'friendly' bacteria in your gut are your first line of defence, and recent research even suggests that pieces of their cell walls can kill cancer cells in *in vitro* tests.

As you go through this book you will come to realise just how much the defence of your body lies in your own hands.

Q6. Are overweight people more prone to cancer?

In early 2003 researchers at the Erasmus Medical Centre in Rotterdam re-analysed an American study involving 3,457 participants aged 30 to 49 and followed over a 42 year period. The results were reported in the *Annals of Internal Medicine*. They concluded that:

- 40 year old male and female non-smokers who were 4–10 kgs over a healthy weight lost 3 years off their life expectancy.
- When the excess exceeded 12 kgs women lost 7 years and men 5.8.
- If they smoked as well, these figures became a loss of 13.5 years.

A second study (*Cancer Epidemology*, Feb 13 2004) concluded that women who gain between 21 and 30 pounds after the age of 18 increase their risks of post-menopausal breast cancer by 40 per cent. If a woman gains over 70 pounds her risk doubles.

Another study concluded that, in general, overweight and obese people are 40 per cent more likely to contract cancer and it is quite easy to see why.

If you eat more, quite simply, you produce more toxic waste products.

If you are overweight you are probably less active, your lymph system stagnates and so the toxins stay in the cellular environment longer.

Often overweight people are overweight because of the types of food they eat. These foods are often high on the list of 'bad foods'. Poor quality eating habits are formed at an early age.

One third of boys under 6 are overweight or obese, rising to almost 50 per cent by the age of 15. Fatty foods and empty calories are destroying these humans early. Fats, fizzy drinks, salted and preserved food, processed quick meals, the list is endless. Parents have a duty to bring their kids up properly and at least half are failing them. Almost half of all children eat no vegetables in a week apart from chips! Recent UK research showed that half of the 10 year olds surveyed could not even identify basic vegetables like cauliflower and broccoli. Schools need to educate the next generation that vegetables are red, green, white and orange and rarely come in fast food cartons.

Food is often prepared in a less than beneficial way. Frying uses oils and fats that give rise to free radical toxins in the body; barbecue-burnt food gives rise to nitrosamines, linked to stomach cancers; and vegetables are often over boiled with loss of vitamins and minerals. Overweight people are often great 'snackers' and many of these foods contain too much sodium (which helps turn cells toxic) and sugar (the favourite food of cancer cells).

Poor eating habits, particularly the consumption of high calorie foods of little nutritional benefit put all people at increased risk of cancer, especially overweight people. The hormones in a healthy body are in a perfect state of balance (homeostasis). Drink lots of fizzy sweet drinks and that all changes instantly because the body produces a surge of insulin to deal with the excess sugar. This then has a knock-on effect to the other hormones in the body and, as we will see in Q19, can negatively influence the cellular environment. Overweight people often eat in such a way (e.g. big meals, high fat meals, lots of sugary foods) that they suddenly flood their bodies with sugar and carbohydrates and these play havoc with their hormones.

And hormones are extremely powerful biochemical substances. A small excess or lack can cause a chain reaction in the body, affecting the immune system and the ability of the body to mop up free radicals, worsening the odds against cancer.

Overweight people also have excess fat stores and fat is a wonderful solvent. It can dissolve, and so hold, more toxins including excess hormones. If an overweight person also fails to encourage lymph movement, the toxins that cannot leave in a dynamic, flowing lymph system will happily be dissolved by the fat cells rendering our fat person extremely toxic, with far higher levels of unwanted hormones, and far more prone to diseases including cancer. A simple case of 'Toxic Waist'!

By contrast, tests on laboratory rats where the calorie count was held at 10 per cent below the normal required daily level, showed 40 per cent increases in life expectancy over the norm.

The evidence is overwhelming. To live longer and to beat cancer? Eat Better. Eat Less.

Q7. How does cancer spread?

The original rogue cell with its unravelled ball of DNA string can simply copy itself repeatedly and rapidly.

Perfect copies of this new rogue cell are made from the original, because the body normally does copy perfectly. So suddenly there are many cells all with the new-look ball of string. Theoretically, if the environment of this poisoned cell is maintained (e.g. if the diet, smoking, sunlight conditions continued) the rogue ball of string becomes the norm in an area of the body.

Meanwhile, the great majority of cells in the body are still in their original state, as is your protective immune system. The healthy immune system should recognise the rogue cells and simply kick them out, if it is strong enough to do so. As we will see later, it has identifier T-cells that look round the body for rogue cells and then bring out the troops to kick them out.

Cancer spreads basically in two ways. The most normal is by the cluster of rogue cells which actively fire cells off into the surrounding lymph or blood systems. However, sometimes the original rogue cell and any copies may also send out messages into the rest of the body. Just as the train read the ball of string and sent a message from the nucleus into the cell, another copy is made in the cell and can be sent in the blood stream throughout the body. This secondary message acts very much like virus and it can poison and decode a recipient cell.

Some rogue cells spread via the blood system to secondary organs like the brain or the liver; some spread via the lymph to lymph nodes. Metastasis is the name given to this process of spreading, and also to the secondary tumours resulting.

However, the fact that hundreds of such messages can be sent out but usually no recipients are infected, means that your body is normally extremely successful in protecting itself. And the fact that cancer sufferers can go into remission or are cured certainly indicates that the body can, **at any time** 'restrengthen' itself and halt the advances of the rogue cells. This is the wondrous power of the immune system.

The issue for everybody is to realise that there are factors that cause cancer and you should do everything in your power to reduce them, whilst also doing everything in your power to boost your immune system. If you are a sufferer already, there are things that are almost certainly 'maintaining' your cancer. For example, if you smoke and the doctor did his best for you in your treatment, you would surely realise that you stand a high chance of the cancer returning if you continued to smoke. So with any cancer ask yourself what might have caused, or be maintaining, it. It is quite possible to reduce the negative causes, boost your immune system and stop the tumour in its tracks. I know a homeopath who did exactly that with her own breast cancer.

Cancer does however possess the ability to hide from our immune system. Not in every case, but sometimes. For example, some tumours can form a 'protein shield' around them making attack very difficult; there are ingredients (like bromelain in pineapple and papain in papaya) in a number of natural foods that help you break down this coat. In other cancers a particular hereditary gene can go wrong on your DNA string. This can prevent the immune system from actually recognizing the rogue cells. Fortunately this is rare (less than seven per cent of people) and where it does happen scientists are already working on new ways of stimulating the immune system into re-recognising the rogues (for example, Dendritic Cell Therapy).

Everybody needs to remember one key phrase 'Love your immune system'; a few people with some hereditary cancer link need to pay special attention to this maxim.

SECTION II

How can I best protect myself
against cancer?

Introduction

Sitting at a table out of doors in regional Thailand I ordered grilled fish. It duly arrived complete with an intact liver, a plate of vegetables and a bowl of steamed rice. I was immediately told that eating the liver would make me clever and keep me from being ill. My partner had steamed chicken (although it was a frugal helping by Western standards) cooked in a 'stew' of lemon grass, galanga and kaffir lime leaves.

The next morning the national newspaper reported that cancer rates in Thailand were expected to double from 60,000 per annum to 120,000 in the next 20 years. The reason for this was laid at the door of the West. Fast food and fried chicken restaurants, coffee and muffin shops have arrived. Thais should get back to basics was the cry; more vegetables, fruit and rice.

In my hotel that morning were a hundred or so overweight and unhealthy looking people, mainly Western tourists. Most were tucking into plate upon plate of ham, eggs, cheese, and bread, toasts and croissants, butter and jam. The more healthy minded (I guess) ate muesli and fibre and a low fat yoghurt; while everyone drank tea and coffee, with or without sugar and milk.

The gym was empty.

My Thai partner had a bowl of rice with some chilli and vegetables followed by fresh fruit. Her drink was water.

The population of the UK is approximately the same as that of Thailand. New cancer cases in the UK this year will approach 270,000.

Q8. How likely am I to contract cancer?

Do you get colds or flu? This may seem a little flippant especially as colds or flu are invasions of the body by external viruses, and in cancer something in the very structure of your body has gone wrong. But the action of the rogue cell in sending out messages inside the body is very like the action of a virus; it's just that the origins are from within. With a normal body 'invaded' by 200 plus rogue cells a day, the immune system is called in to play, whether it is a cancer attack or a flu attack. This is why it is important to 'love your immune system'.

Similarly, just as there are many strains of 'cold' or of 'flu', there is no one single cancer. Tumours take many forms, have many starting points and are as individual as you are. Two people diagnosed with the same cancer can have very different causal and biochemical relationships with it. This will affect its growth and their ability to beat it. This is why you do hear such wonderful stories of people 'curing' themselves, whilst others try everything with little success. There is a great deal that every cancer sufferer can do to improve their odds of a cure. There's also a great deal we can all do to prevent a cancer taking hold.

As I said in the introduction, on current statistics two out of three people will not contract cancer. And of cancer sufferers, three quarters will beat it. There are many things you can do to increase the odds, specifically strengthening your immune system and avoiding the pitfalls. As we shall see, you are a complex mixture of hormones, immune and body energy systems, all of which can be boosted to aid your defence. Think positively, be disciplined and realise that, despite the growing worldwide statistics, **you can build your own little micro-environment of health**. You can increase your odds.

The worldwide statistics on cancer are awesome. It has reached epidemic proportions. After car accidents, leukaemia and brain tumours are the second and third biggest causes of death in children in the Western world. In the next 30 years at least one in eight women will have breast cancer and one in three men over 60 will be diagnosed with prostate cancer. In fact, there are over 200 other forms of cancer including, just for example, lung

33

cancer, skin cancer, stomach and colon cancer, liver and pancreatic cancer.

Four out of 10 people in the UK will be diagnosed with cancer.

Worse still, the rates are increasing. Macmillan Cancer Relief predict rates will triple by 2025 in the UK. And it is now estimated that, of Americans born today, one in two will develop cancer.

In the UK, childhood cancers are 30 per cent higher than 45 years ago, germ cell tumours are 50 per cent higher, brain cancer is up 36 per cent and acute lymphoblastic leukaemia is up 33 per cent. The figures do not make good reading. If these were road or flying accidents there would be an outcry, a major overhaul on safety and an examination of the causes. Not so with cancer.

Against this background, an increasing concern is 'over diagnosis'. Prostate cancer and breast cancer are two cancers rapidly growing in the Western world, but some experts are now questioning whether the figures are what they seem. In May 2004 the Institute for Cancer Research published an 11 year study of 'active surveillance' from the Royal Marsden. It concluded that as many as 50 per cent of men diagnosed with prostate cancer did not need invasive treatment! A survey of men aged over 50 killed in road accidents in Los Angeles showed almost half were driving around blissfully ignorant of their disease. Digital Rectal Examinations and PSA tests, are notoriously inaccurate at identifying prostate cancer.

For women, the recent Breast Cancer Conferences in San Diego (2003) and Europe (2004) were illuminating. Mammograms were stated to be, at best, 67 per cent accurate. In 50 per cent of cases they indicated DCIS, which is actually not cancer but calcified deposits in breast ducts. At UCLA they are warning that only about 20 per cent of these will ever lead to cancer and so referring to them as cancers or precancers is grossly misleading. Vitamin D can help reduce such calcification.

Both men and women need to be absolutely certain that their cancer is proven and understand what are the risks of leaving it alone, and not just treating it because a 'threat' is there! Unfortunately the medical world seems wound-up in a 'treat-it-early' frenzy and urgent panic action is just not necessary in a number of cases.

For most people two factors contribute to the fact that 80 per cent of all cancers hit those people over the age of 60:

- **A slow steady build up of toxins as a by-product of our normal daily lives**
- **A natural age related decline in our defensive hormone and immune systems.**

Sir Richard Doll and Sir Richard Peto of Oxford University looked at the causes of cancer in a study funded by the Imperial Cancer Research Fund and the Medical Research Council. They concluded that, for example:

35% cancers were caused	by diet
30% "	by smoking
10% "	by reproductive hormones
10% "	by infection
5% "	by alcohol.

They also concluded that only a very small percentage are due to environmental factors or pollution and up to 2 per cent of cancers are caused by some sort of virus, bacterium, parasite or yeast. These figures are now known to be much too small and, again, they completely ignored factors associated with mental state such as stress.

If cancer involves a very complex multi-stage process only rarely can it be caused by just one factor, so the above figures seem a bit too black and white to me. Although factors like asbestos and extreme sunshine may cause the whole chain re-action of cancer formation, people are most at risk when hit by several factors, for example, those on a poor diet, who are over-weight, smoke, and drink. The odds increase disproportionately the more hits you have.

The above study also seems to fail to fully integrate the role of all environmental factors into this complex process. Clearly air and water impurity, toxin residues in foods, toxins in household products, toiletries and cosmetic products, prescription medi-cines, and pesticides must all be shaping our overall lives and our health. For example, the WWF has produced several studies showing that we all have a number of known toxins (from DDT

35

to PCB's and even flame retardants) in our blood streams and that our children have almost double the levels of their grand-parents.

To date, the majority of cancers appear to be a more Western lifestyle phenomenon. For instance, breast and prostate cancers are virtually non-existent in China and Thailand, whilst Japan runs at a quarter of the rate in Britain. Even people in Nagasaki and Hiroshima, those sites of nuclear explosions, are only a fifth as likely to get a prostate or breast cancer as people living in the West.

In the 1950s and 60s breast cancer was rare in Japan but the more affluent Japanese women have now forsaken their original, mainly vegetarian rice and vegetable diets to follow a more Western diet of dairy products and meat with alarming conse-quences. Age adjusted mortality rates in Japan show that in the 30 years from 1968, breast cancer in women and kidney cancer in men have both doubled, whilst kidney cancer in women, brain cancers generally and multiple myeloma have increased by over 300 per cent. The Heidelberg Cancer Research Centre found that vegetarians have more than twice the immune defence ability to knock out cancer cells than non-vegetarians.

Since so few cancers can actually be completely cured by the official medical establishment despite billions of dollars being spent on drug development, the crucial issue is not to contract it in the first place. Published data in the USA shows that apart from major advances in the cure rates of cancers such as testicu-lar and childhood leukaemia, the overall cure rate in the last 10 years is virtually static. UK statistics show cancer has increased by almost 4 per cent per annum for the last 25 years, whilst five-year survival has increased by only 12 per cent in 30 years, or 0.4 per cent per annum.

If all this doesn't start a sensible argument for the creation of a serious cancer prevention body there are many hundreds of further facts beyond the scope of this book that complete the picture. This is exactly why we have formed CANCERactive. Every one of us is vulnerable and we need a good honest appraisal of our lifestyles, our environment, the products we use and our diets. If you have cancer, clean up your act!!

Where possible a more back-to-basics approach to living will help, but even that may not be enough with the tide of possible cancer causes flooding our way.

Cancer sufferers often ask themselves: 'Why me?' In fact all non-sufferers should be asking: 'Why not me?'

Q9. What can we learn from cancer sufferers?

When someone has cancer it is a 'must' to look beyond the tumour to the possible causes and elements that are sustaining it. For the sufferer this increases the odds of a cure. But for the non-sufferer it is enormously helpful too. There are generally four factors common to cancer sufferers:

(i)   Cancer sufferers are 'toxic', as we have discussed
(ii) Cancer sufferers often have 'acid' cells
(iii) Cancer sufferers often have a parasite (and/or heavy yeast infection) and about 20 per cent have some sort of virus
(iv) Cancer sufferers can have a self-debilitating mental attitude.

You will note I have not included 'heredity'. This is because of the Swedish research amongst identical twins that I mentioned earlier; that even with similar genes there is much you can do in your diet, attitude, and lifestyle to prevent a cancer occurring. You just have to try harder and take more care!

(i) Toxins

Throughout this book we will mention toxins, be they chemical, tobacco or diet related. Toxins pervade the bloodstream, the lymph and get into cells where they do their damage. We will also talk about how you can avoid the toxins and/or expel them from your system by factors like having a good diet, or by drinking clean water, ensuring healthy bowel movements or through detoxing and cleaning your liver.

(ii) Acid bodies

One of the basic ways we all make our cells toxic is through our day-in-day-out Western diets.

As we have seen, a variety of observers believe 35 to 50 per cent of cancers are caused by diet.

The fact is that our bodies work best when they are slightly alkaline. Our immune system works best at an alkaline pH as do our cells. Unfortunately, we make our cells acid.

A prime culprit is 'salt'. We eat too much sodium and not enough potassium and magnesium. (A much more detailed explanation and solution can be found in *The Tree of Life: The Anti-Cancer Diet*.)

Over the hundreds of thousands of years we developed as humans our cells, and particularly their power stations, built a system of energy production based around chemical reactions using potassium. If you eat too much sodium it displaces the potassium making the energy production less efficient and using less oxygen. The sodium makes the power stations more acid too. Acidity, poor performance, low oxygen – these are the precursors of a cancer cell. Sodium is typically found in salt and sea salt, meat preservatives, monosodium glutamate and especially in prepared and procesed foods.

Magnesium – and a recent US survey showed 40 per cent of Americans were deficient in magnesium – helps a pump on every cell push potassium into the cell and kick out sodium.

Moreover, all foodstuffs can be divided into those that leave an alkaline residue and those that leave an acid one; our modern lifestyle and diet pushes us towards the acid producing foods containing sodium or those producing sulphur by-products, for example meats and fish, whereas our forefathers 100 years or more ago had an alkaline producing diet.

From various sources I have compiled a gradient of acidity such that acid residue 'beware' is minus 5 points; 'extremely acid' is minus 4 points; 'very acid' minus 3; 'moderately acid' minus 2 and 'slightly acid' minus 1. Alkaline residue producers are given plus points, up to a maximum of 4. (See Tables I and II.)

How well do you do in a day?

As you can see there are not that many high yield alkaline producers. (For a full list of acid and alkaline residue producers, see appendix I.)

You can buy pH testing kits to measure your body's acidity and you can have your blood and cellular biochemistry analysed to check your levels of stress, your vitamin and mineral content, your allergies and intolerances (see Vega later).

If you are too acid correct by (i) changing your diet to cut out acid residue foods; (ii) cutting sodium and adding in potassium

Table I Acid Producers – some examples	
Liver, crab, shellfish, scallops, stress	-5
All meats, lack of sleep, fried foods	-4
Most fish, eggs, crisps, peanuts and similar snacks, processed meats and smoked fish, sauces, vinegars, mustards, chocolate, salt, spirits, white wine, cigarettes.	-3
Most refined wheat based products, fizzy soft drinks, oranges, tomatoes, refined rice, noodles, pasta, coffee, tea, dairy, red wine.	-2
Lentils, chickpeas, dried beans, beer, whole wheat, bananas, prunes, plums.	-1

Table II Alkaline Producers – some examples	
Apples, pears, all green vegetables, cranberries, fresh nuts, melons, pumpkin, onions, oats, millet, rye, asparagus.	+1
All berries, cherries, mangoes, lychees, coconut, peaches, grapes, carrots potatoes, parsnips, turnips, fresh beetroot, lemons, watercress, papaya, whole brown rice, soya beans and soya.	+2
Garlic, kale, dates and figs especially dried, raisins	+3
Cooked spinach, noni juice, fresh ginger.	+4

and magnesium rich foods; (iii) taking coral calcium or carctol (Q20), both excellent alkalisers.

(iii) Parasites, yeasts, viruses, and bacteria

Parasites

People tend to think of parasites as quite large organisms like tapeworms or liver flukes, but in Carolina over 80 per cent of the population has a parasite. It is microscopic and comes from the water system; it is immune to chlorine. Other microscopic parasites can take up residence having arrived on your fruit.

In one report a doctor in Boston found that 42 of his thousand or so patients had liver fluke and, on killing the parasite, their cancer condition improved markedly. **In another study 80 per cent of cancer patients were found to have a parasite.** Some UK practitioners believe that most, if not all, of their cancer patients have some sort of parasite. Worryingly, since 1997 levels of fluke have quadrupled in British livestock according to government figures.

One reason for the rising incidence of parasites in the USA is felt to be their increased transmission through sexual activity (even simply kissing an infected host). Another is the parasites' diminished requirement for a secondary host in order to survive. All parasites historically have needed at least two hosts. Now it is felt that certain ingested solvents and pollutants like isopropyl alcohol, a by-product from contaminants of animal fat, pesticides and hygiene products, allow some flukes to multiply in just one host. Certainly isopropyl alcohol and aflatoxin B seem to be found in large quantities if a parasite is present and this creates a carcinogenic environment for the host.

Aflatoxin B seems to be produced by certain parasites and is highly toxic. Linus Pauling, the champion of vitamin C, claimed that large doses in excess of one gram of vitamin C a day would have a positive effect on some cancer sufferers. One possible explanation is that vitamin C has been found to neutralise aflatoxin B.

Yeasts
A very common phenomenon in the Western world is yeast infection. In developing nations where you think parasites and yeasts would have more hold over the population, a review of local diets shows a prevalence of food stuffs like chilli, garlic, cinnamon, cloves, fennel and oregano, or natural additives like bee propolis, Pau d'Arco, wormwood or neem, all of which keep yeasts in check in the body.

In the West, however, we eat few of these 'preventers' and take steroids, antibiotics and even chemotherapy all of which kill the friendly bacteria in our bodies. Each night when you sleep these 'good guys' devour the yeasts and the microbes in your intestine. If you've destroyed your 'good guys' you've little defence and the yeasts multiply.

Rather like mushrooms, they have a matrix of fine roots, which go across the gut lining and into the blood supply. This can allow toxins to pass straight from your stomach to your blood. Worse, eventually yeasts can pass into the bloodstream and round the body, where they 'collonise' around healthy cells. Yeasts do not use oxygen to create their life energy, so the environment they create is oxygen-free – exactly the environment that favours cancer cells.

Again much more in terms of action you can take, can be found on this in *The Tree of Life: The Anti-Cancer Diet* and on our website: www.iconmag.co.uk

It is estimated that up to 70 per cent of the UK population has an over-development of yeasts.

The effect of both parasites and yeasts is similar. They deplete the body of nourishment and vitamins, and especially B vitamins, whilst increasing the level of toxins in the host's body and weakening their immune system.

Viruses

Up to 20 per cent of people are thought to have some sort of long-term viral infection. The herpes virus is now being linked to some vaginal and prostate cancers. Experts at Pittsburg University have found a statistical link between prostate cancer and people with the cold sore virus. There are nine types of herpes virus, only one being passed sexually. Others include shingles, chicken pox and glandular fever. Indeed some cases of breast cancer appear to follow an attack of shingles.

There is a link between human papilloma virus (HPV) and several cancers but, in particular, cervical cancer. Viruses are also linked to cancers of the liver and blood.

The whole issue of viruses causing cancer was 'put on ice' about 30 years ago and other cancer issues took priority. Now with better analytical techniques there is a move to study this subject in depth. You can expect to hear more and more about viral causes of cancer. It may well be that certain viral infections are causal; it may also be that people with weaker immune systems are more likely to get cancer and viral infections (i.e. it is purely co-incidence); either way the pharmaceutical companies are extremely interested. Vaccinating whole populations is big business!

Already some scientists are arguing that viruses may well cause 40 per cent of all cancers. At the MD Anderson Cancer Centre in Houston, Texas the Simian Virus (Monkey Virus, SV40) turned up in 33 out of 55 cases of Hodgkin's lymphoma. Other seats of learning are worried about the same virus and have tried to link it to other cancers such as brain tumours. Again viral infection robs the host of nourishment, increases levels of toxins and weakens the immune system, often in quite a localised area.

Bacteria

The relatively common bacterium helicobacter pylori, which only recently was linked to stomach ulcers, is now being associated with stomach cancer. It can be eliminated using a cocktail of antibiotics, or simply by taking Goldenseal and bismuth. Similar bacterial infections are also linked to bladder cancer.

Chlamydia is another sexually transmitted bacterial infection, and research evidence links this to ovarian cancer and also to some cervical cancers.

Human Papilloma Virus (HPV)

HPV is the fastest spreading sexually transmitted disease. Usually the virus is simply cleared out of the body in a year or so, although in some cases it may remain dormant for a very long time. More than half of all sexually active Americans will carry the virus at some point in their lives. Men are unlikely to even know they have it.

HPV enters through tiny abrasions in the skin and condoms are not much use as mere skin contact is usually enough to pass on the virus. No reliable tests exist and there is currently no treatment or cure.

Worse it is a 'smart' virus and even the immune system does not seem to notice its presence because it multiplies prodigiously inside a skin cell, which then dies. These dead skin cells are literally virus 'pods' ready to spread to the next host.

HPV causes cervical cancer, cancers of the genitalia and anus and is implicated in several others.

To put figures on this about 500,000 women worldwide contract cervical cancer each year and only 50 per cent survive five years.

Vaccines are being developed, and one by Merck Sharpe and Dohme and a similar product from Glaxo are in final trials now. They seem effective with two strains of HPV that account for 70 per cent of cervical cancers. However such vaccines are preventative and have no effect if the man or woman is already a carrier. Such preventative vaccines also bring with them a debate over at what age people should be vaccinated, particularly as the age at which first sexual contact takes place is reducing.

Although the medical world says there is no way of detecting HPV presence, some homeopaths believe they can detect it, and this may be a route to explore if you are concerned. Indeed, some homeopaths also believe they can eradicate HPV from the body.

For the moment the best answer seems to be long-term monogamy!

The important point is that many seemingly normal people may well be carriers of parasites, yeasts or viruses and need to deal with them. It is possible to be tested for many viruses, parasites and yeast and bacteria, by homeopaths and specialist cancer clinics. (See Q32.)

Where cancer sufferers are concerned it is **imperative** that tests are carried out to see if they are infected, so that these 'enemies of the state' can be eradicated quickly if they are detected.

Many viruses can be treated using modern drugs. Parasites can be eradicated over time :

• By taking steps to cleanse your diet (e.g. using clean and filtered water, by removing uncooked meats and dairy products from your diet)

44

- By avoiding certain pollutants, e.g. isopropyl alcohol from personal products and pesticides
- By taking a number of natural products to remove the parasites or their toxic by-products, e.g. a mixture of natural ingredients like ground cloves, wormwood, garlic, ginger, anise and slippery elm with vitamin C (there are proprietary products you can buy).

Yeasts can be treated by using garlic, Pau d'Arco, caprylic acid, wormwood and oregano and by adopting an alcohol, dairy, sugar and yeasty food (Marmite, mushrooms, etc) free diet. Again proprietary brands can be used. Yeast sufferers should also take acidophilus tablets in high strength form. (This is no bad thing for everybody. The stomach can lose its complete supply of good bacteria in just three days if you are unwell.)

In all three cases the immune system should be boosted with zinc 15 mgs, vitamin C 1 gm (take as four times 250 gms across the day) and B complex (especially biotin 0.3 mgs). It is also crucial that both partners, for example a husband and wife where one has cancer, take the anti-parasite treatment since otherwise it might just pass back and forward between them.

Even if yeasts, parasites, and viruses do not actually cause cancer they do play their part in weakening the whole immune system by increasing toxins and removing vitamins. This makes the body much more vulnerable to contracting or sustaining cancer. Sadly, modern medicine pays little attention to any of these possible contributory factors despite the latest findings of the scientists.

As an example of the influence of yeasts, Pau d'Arco for a long time was thought to have great anti-cancer benefits. But it is now thought that this is more likely to be due to the indirect effect of killing off yeasts rather than any direct effect on cancer cells.

However, interestingly, wormwood has been shown to also have anti-cancer properties.

(iv) A self-debilitating mental attitude

This is a huge subject and the reason why a whole section of this book (section III) is devoted to 'mind over matter'.

Cancer sufferers are often the nicest people but they are not being true to themselves. They like to please others and put others first, often neglecting their own well-being. They don't like to trouble people. Because of such emotional factors like strong feelings of guilt or unworthiness, they seek peer group approval and put up with unhappy jobs or unhappy surroundings (including people who put them down). As a result they often live in environments that just don't 'fit', they neglect their own true happiness and they have little sense of purpose or emotional reward. Often they simply put up with undue stresses and problems because they feel it is their lot.

Their inability to be true to themselves is linked to a lowered self-esteem and self-worth. They do not take time for themselves and this leads to greater imbalances between the life they lead and the life they need, at emotional and physical levels. As Section III will show, this directly leads to a reduced body energy level and a measurable decline in the immune system of up to 30 per cent.

Everybody should put themselves through an emotional and physical 'health check' regularly and ask what makes them happy, what makes them unhappy, what causes most stress. Defining a sense of purpose that would fulfil them, planning a lifestyle that provides time for mental and physical 'nourishment', relaxation and stimulation and removing the creators of toxins (including people) that influence their lives.

Depression has strong links to cancer. Depression lowers oxygen levels in the blood and cells by up to 30 per cent (and thus cancer, which hates oxygen, can thrive).

Depression also affects the cellular environment negatively through the eicosanoid system (see Q19) and it is no wonder that depression alone has been linked to 30 to 40 per cent of all cancers. *Time* magazine in January 2003 carried a thorough scientific review.

Q10. Which environmental carcinogens may cause cancer?

'It isn't pollution that's harming the environment. It's the impurities in our air and water that's doing it'. These words of wisdom were provided by none less a person than the former Vice-President of the USA, Dan Quayle.

As said before, the onset of cancerous cells is a multi-step process and that environmental, lifestyle and diet issues individually are usually not enough to cause cancer. Predisposition and infection are also co-factors. However, let's start with a look at some of the environmental factors that we come into contact with almost every day. I do not want to labour any of these points, just give you a brief picture.

(i) Water

'Even the Archbishop of Canterbury is 80 per cent water', said J B Haldane a notable biochemist more than half a century ago. Water is vital to all our bodily functions, the provision of fuels to our cells and the removal of waste and toxins. Athletes or people in extreme terrains who have a 10 per cent fall in their hydration level experience a 50 per cent fall in everything from their energy levels to their ability to concentrate.

Tap water, depending upon your location, can have a mixture of parasites, heavy and toxic metals like copper and lead from the pipes, pesticides, nitrites, and aluminium from the water purification process, oestrogen, and even radioactivity. In some places the level of chlorine at certain times of the day can exceed levels recommended for swimming pools. Chlorine can change the body's pH and kill the friendly bacteria essential for intestinal health.

Oestrogen is a particularly worrying component in recycled tap waters. Caused by the increased use of the birth control pill and HRT, some lakes and rivers have been shown to have a disproportionate number of female fish, with male fish losing their male characteristics. Certainly changing diets and factors such as oestrogen consumption have seen a change in the ratio of boys to girls born in the UK. A hundred years ago more boys were born, but now this has been reversed. There is also concern that oestrogen and chemicals which mimic oestrogen in our tap waters is a factor in causing human sperm counts to fall.

Boiling the water doesn't help much as this merely serves to concentrate some of the metals and pollutants. (You would need to distil the water rather than simply boil it, but nutrients would then be lost).

Bottled water also has its problems, as plastic bottles are known to leach out carcinogens (phthalates, which are oestrogen mimics) into the water. Far safer is water in glass bottles.

Most water filters are quite good, but they are limited in their effectiveness. One possible solution is a serious reverse osmosis water filter, but even some of those can be ineffective with oestrogen, and the irony is the water produced is slightly acid and is felt by some people to be too clean!

(ii) Silent killers?

Radiation
The Royal College of Radiologists believes that as many as 250 cases of fatal cancers are caused each year by X-rays. Professor Gofman of UCLA believes that as many as 75 per cent of breast cancers are actually caused by medical X-rays in the USA. X-rays during pregnancy have been directly linked to a 50 per cent increase in childhood leukaemia.

CAT scans give you a much higher dose of radiation than normal X-rays, whilst MRI scans subject the body to forces 50,000 times those normally encountered on earth. Recent Canadian research has concluded that people having an annual CT scan have a one-in-fifty risk of death! 'The dangers are well known', said the professor in charge of the project (**icon** – November 2004). Research is currently underway to see if MRI scans can cause cancer.

Mammograms are the subject of huge debate. They provide approximately 1,000 times the dose of an X-ray.

Dense breast tissue is risky breast tissue and is linked to breast cancer. Unfortunately Western women's high levels of oestrogen, coupled with diet and lifestyle, results in dense tissue. However, the denser the tissue the less likely a mammogram is to spot an early developing tumour. It is a serious conundrum facing doctors and all women in the West. A safer system is on the way. About four locations in the UK use non-invasive, non-damaging and highly accurate thermal imaging. The University of Southern California (Perisley 2003) quotes their studies that infra-red imagining is 99 per cent accurate. Sadly the medical profession is financially committed to offering mamograms. The hospitals already have the expensive machinery!

Radiation from medical treatments is also a concern. Interestingly, the health correspondent of *The Times* in November 2002, seeking to play down fears of the damage caused by a dirty terrorist bomb which would scatter radiation dust in the air, claimed it was only similar to the dose from a whole body X-ray. If true this would make a mammogram as 'dirty' as 1,000 Al Qaeda bombs!

Electromagnetic fields (EMFs)
Every one of us has a natural body energy field around us and it can be dangerous and unhealthy to interfere with this. Dr Reiter of the University of Texas, San Antonio, leads a team of researchers who have linked EMFs to the suppression of melatonin production and to an increased cancer risk.

Nine studies in the UK show that relatively low levels of EMFs from power cables, pylons or mains electricity are directly linked to an increased risk of childhood cancer, especially leukaemia. This has been confirmed in the USA and Sweden.

What of sockets either side of the bed head, TVs in the bedroom or electric blankets? All can be unwanted sources of localised EMFs.

It would be wise to reduce your exposure to TV and VDU screens. TVs should be 3 metres away from the viewer as a minimum and covered from view in a bedroom at night, even if they are switched off. VDUs should always be switched off when not in use and less powerful alternatives, for example, powerbooks, used where possible.

And it is possible to live on dangerous fault lines of electromagnetic energy. Transmitters on hills can have magnetic fields lying between them, causing hot spots.

In January 2002 the small Spanish village of Valladolid won a landmark victory to remove 36 mobile phone transmitters installed on a building 50 metres from the local primary school.

In the 18 months since the masts had been erected four of the children had developed cancer, yet prior to it there had not been a case for 34 years.

Other houses have quite unexplained magnetic fields running through them, which appear not to be linked to power lines or to have geological sources. Dr Clarke of the UK Radiological Protection Board was quoted as saying: '*It could be the way the homes were wired or something about their supply, or their use of appliances.*'

Mobile phones

If you turn a phone on and it is making a call, when you place it next to a bucket of water 90 per cent of the phone's ionising radiation will pass into the bucket of water. This phenomenon is called induction. In fact, only a small proportion of the power of a mobile phone is actually used in transmitting the call to the receiver mast; the rest goes into any nearby object, your head, your hand, your hips.

Dr Lennart Hardel has released two papers (the last in October 2002 – *International Journal of Radiation Biology*), linking mobile phones with malignant brain tumours. A third paper by Mild, another Swedish researcher, in 2003 concluded that people using a mobile phone, or a cordless house phone, for over one hour a day had a 30 per cent increased risk of a brain tumour.

The Finnish Radiation and Nuclear Safety Authority has reported its view that mobile phones caused activity in the cells lining the blood-brain barrier changing its ability to protect the brain from harmful substances.

Colorado University researchers have shown that frequent mobile phone users had significantly depressed melatonin levels (see Q18).

The Environmental Health Trust concludes, '*20–80 per cent of the electromagnetic radiation generated by mobile phones (depend-*

ing upon the make) is directly absorbed into the user's brain.' And, *'A few minutes exposure to cell-phone type radiation can transform a 5 per cent active cancer into a 95 per cent active cancer'.*

Around 25 per cent of mobile phones are used by the under 18s, and according to a report in *The Ecologist*, children are most in danger because their skulls are thinner, allowing the radiation to penetrate further into their brains. With a developing nervous system they are more prone to memory impairment and immune deficiency. A recent Spanish research study confirms this. A child using a mobile phone, even for a very short period, experiences a significant slowing of brain function for up to 50 minutes.

Roger Coghill, an anti-mobile phone biologist has recently been defeated in his case to have warning labels introduced. But he is quite clear, *'Anyone who uses a mobile phone for longer than 20 minutes quite literally should have their head examined'.*

Radon
Radon is a radioactive gas formed by the natural radioactive decay of uranium in rock, soil and water. Low levels of uranium occur widely in the earth's crust and some areas have more than others.

Radon itself is colourless, tasteless, odourless and chemically inert. Unless you test for it, you'd never know it was there. Once produced by the uranium, it bubbles up through the ground into the air above.

The problem comes if you are in a higher-than-average radon area. Radon accumulates inside homes, building up to high levels that are not easily dispersed. Electrically charged atoms from the radon attach themselves to dust particles, which can be inhaled. Inside your lungs the decaying particles produce radiation, which has the potential to damage lung tissue.

The Surgeon General in the USA has warned that radon is the second leading cause of lung cancer and is a 'serious public health problem'. (*National Academy of Sciences*). It is estimated that 40,000 cases of lung cancer are caused each year in the USA by radon. Problem areas in the UK include Wales and the South West, but there are pockets in the Midlands, north of Manchester and north east of Edinburgh.

There is also evidence of a synergistic effect between radon and smoking, which increases risk by 55 per cent, (*National Safety Council, Washington*).

If you are worried about radon or lung cancer, you can get your home checked. (Details in appendix II.)

Gas appliances
Although there is absolutely no evidence to link gas appliances to cancer, there is concern that exhaust products from them weaken the immune system and have been linked, for example, to arthritis. Levels of nitrogen dioxide in homes with gas boilers and gas cookers may exceed government levels laid down as constituting severe pollution in city environments.

Diesel fumes
Diesel fumes cause similar problems to radon. The fumes are particulate, and the 'nasties' can be inhaled into the deepest corners of your lungs. US research is quite clear about the links to lung cancer. Recent research has shown a four-fold incidence of leukaemia in children living near petrol stations. The exact cause is unknown (**icon** – November 2004)

Chemical pollution
In the 1930's the world produced 1 million tonnes of chemicals. Now that figure is 400 million tonnes. The WWF has conducted several studies with a list of some of the most toxic like pesticides and PCB's. Sadly, of the 78 most potent, on average we each have 29 in our blood streams in the UK. Pesticides can be avoided by choosing organic food or growing your own. But, by and large, our chemical exposure is outside our hands. Except that our in-home use of cleaners and household products makes pollution in the home actually higher than in Times Square according to US research. See 'Safe as Houses' on www.iconmag.co.uk for information on how you can clean up your home.

(iii) Medicines, antibiotics, anti-inflammatories and vaccines

In their book *Brain Fitness*, Dr Robert Goldman and Dr Ronald Klatz, the President of the American Academy of Anti-Ageing

Medicine, define both antibiotics and anti-inflammatories as 'brain poisons'. The *Journal of the American Medical Association* (Feb 18, 2004) reported on a study of 10,000 women showing those who had taken antibiotics for more than 500 days during a 17 year period had more than twice the risk of breast cancer. Whether this is a direct toxic effect, or an indirect effect (for example, by encouraging high yeast levels in the body) is not clear.

A leading US authority (Moore) claimed that prescription drugs pose the largest group of avoidable toxins available to Americans. Another survey of 240 high usage US prescription drugs stated that over half contained known carcinogens and posed serious risk of cancer at normal dosage levels. Many drugs have not been around long enough for us to know what their long-term effect as carcinogens is likely to be.

Why not go to a cranial osteopath, homeopath or acupuncturist next time you are ill? No one ever said these people could cause cancer and they may well find an underlying reason for the problem, a solution which may not require antibiotics or drugs in the long term.

Vaccinations are a cause for some concern, particularly as there have been no in-depth studies on their safety in relation to cancer. The arguments are based on the toxic way the vaccines are prepared, the impurities contained such as mercury, and the chance of the viruses used in the vaccines themselves causing cancer.

Even the vitamin industry is not immune to selling us carcinogens. Some multivitamins and minerals in pill form can contain toxic heavy metals, whilst some mass produced fish oils, especially from fish caught in coastal waters, can contain dioxins.

(iv) Over exposure to sunlight

Many cancer institutes, including our own Cancer Research UK, believe that strong sunlight seems able to provide all the multistep processes in cancer formation, particularly in people who take white bodies for a two-week trip to the sun. Unfortunately, the research 'evidence' is clouded but sunscreens may not give us the protection we had hoped; some have recently been banned in

53

Scandanavian countries for containing carcinogenic ingredients. P.A.B.A. has been implicated in cancer and should be avoided.

Women using the contraceptive pill have double the risk of melanoma when exposed to the sun. This oestrogen link almost certainly extends to the oestrogen-mimic effect of some chemicals in sunscreens (including their perfumes and preservatives such as parabens) and probably shows that our rapidly increasing levels of skin cancer and melanoma in the UK are not just simply the result of more sun but due to the fact that we are more pre-sensitised than in the past. In fact the most recent research (*Journal of Nat. Cancer Inst*, 2005, 99) supports this casting serious doubt on the over-simplistic view that 'sun is bad'. At the Karolinska Institute in Sweden good sun exposure was shown to reduce levels of skin cancers; one, Non-Hodgkins by up to 40%. In New Mexico high levels of sun were associated with lowered levels of melanoma, almost certainly due to the protective effects of vitamin D produced when sunlight metabolises the cholesterol levels under our white skins.

Until someone comes up with the definitive study beware of perfumed sunscreens containing P.A.B.A. or parabens and avoid over-exposure especially at the start of a trip, particularly lying in the sun in hot countries between 11am and 3pm.

People should be wary of sunbeds too. Professor Andrew Tannahill, chief executive officer of the Health Education Board for Scotland says, *'Weekly use exposes people to six times the annual dose of UV radiation. Sunbeds have always been suspected of causing skin cancer. The evidence is now clear.'*

(v) Insecticides and pesticides

Pesticides have been implicated in many illnesses ranging from birth defects to cancer. The link between cancer and pesticide exposure is well documented. Again, many pesticides act inside the body as chemical oestrogen mimics. Pesticides used at home, for example, to kill flies, on dog collars and to eradicate garden insects, links to a four-fold increase in childhood leukaemia and a greater incidence of brain tumours. Children under 14 whose gardens are sprayed with herbicides have a four times greater incidence of connective tissue tumours.

Some commercial apple trees are sprayed 10–12 times. After picking, apples are waxed so that they look good in shops. It is then virtually impossible to wash the residue of the pesticides off the apple skin. Broccoli, a wonderful source of vitamins C and E, glucosinolates and indole 3 carbinol, collects pesticide under the florets making washing it out equally difficult. In 2004 the UK Soil Association published a scientific review on pesticides and organic food. This prompted Sir John Krebs, Chairman of the Food Standards Agency, to admit for the first time that organic foods did indeed have less pesticides in them. One study reviewed showed that women with breast cancer were five times more likely to have pesticides in their blood than healthy women.

Many pesticides actually mimic the action of oestrogen once in the body. DDT and Lindane are two such culprits and are still found in the food chain in imported foods.

The US Natural Resources Defence Council in their 1989 report concluded that eight pesticides in particular, commonly used on fruit and vegetables, and regularly consumed by pre-school children, made them more likely to develop cancer later in life.

There are believed to be high residues of many carcinogens in fruits, grains and vegetables, yet there is little legislation, and health warnings are not apparent.

Only recently the US Environmental Protection Agency's estimate of the amount of such residues you can safely consume in a lifetime was shown to be exceeded by a baby's total consumption in its first year of life.

This is made more acute by the finding that the young have a much higher susceptibility to carcinogens than their parents do. Tests on young mice show as much as 100 per cent mortality with carcinogens that have no effect on the parents. There are also very real concerns about the consumption of carcinogens by pregnant women and the long-term effects on the unborn child.

(vi) Air quality

Oxygen is the enemy of cancer. At school we learned that air is 21 per cent oxygen. Several hundred thousand years ago this figure was over 30 per cent. In polluted cities it can be as low as 12 per cent and life ceases below 7 per cent.

To beat cancer you need clean, efficient lungs taking in clean, oxygenated air. Most of us compound the problem of poor air quality because we simply do not breathe properly, taking short, almost superficial breaths from chest movements rather than deep breaths using our diaphragms. As a result, stagnant air collects in the lower third to half of our lungs leaving them full of toxins that need to be expelled to avoid our systems being polluted. The action of yawning is caused by this stagnation and the polluted body feeling tired and listless. An external pollutant like carbon monoxide from exhausts and cigarettes, makes matters worse; not only does it take up space in your lungs but it binds with the haemoglobin, reducing its ability to carry oxygen to the cells.

Everybody, as a minimum, needs to spend time going for energetic walks in the countryside, avoiding polluted places and taking time to breathe fresh air deeply. Early morning light exercise, ideally in fresh air and using deep breaths, does you good. It is interesting that an important part of the Chinese approach to cancer therapy involves deep breathing exercises.

(vii) Toxins in household products, toiletries, and cosmetics

Carcinogens surround us and are contained in everything from toothpaste to shampoos, and household cleaners to mouth-washes. Most plastic packaging contains carcinogens that leach out into the food and liquid.

In 1995 David Steinman and Samuel Epstein co-wrote *The Safe Shoppers Bible*. This book is awesome in its review of 4,000 US consumer products including household products, cosmetic, toiletries, and food detailing lists of carcinogenic ingredients.

Epstein is also chairman of the Cancer Prevention Coalition in the USA and worked with Ralph Nader to name and shame the 'Dirty Dozen' consumer products. In 1995 he named toxic ingredients in a number of products including some household cleaners, talcum powder (directly linked to ovarian cancer), permanent hair colour, make-up, a weed killer, toothpaste, and a hair conditioner. In 2001 he wrote a book entitled *Unreasonable Risk*, listing two pages of carcinogens found in US cosmetic and personal care products, of which 40 actually feature on labels (open ingredients) whilst 30 are hidden. Even in the open category, seven are proven 'genotoxins' i.e. in animal or human studies they have been shown to induce genetic damage and the mainstream petrochemical industry admits there is no way of determining thresholds or safety levels. Over the last five years just a few concerns recorded in the press have been:

- Sodium lauryl sulphate (SLS) and sodium laureth sulphate are skin irritants, the latter less so. They can damage eyes and whilst not carcinogenic themselves, they can cause chemical interaction with other ingredients. Of most significance is that SLS increases the permeability of the skin by up to 40 per cent, allowing more chemical toxins into the body. These two compounds are regularly found in soaps, shampoos, toothpastes and body washes.
- Many toothpastes contain sodium fluoride, which in concentrated form is more normally associated with rat poison. Toothpaste packs in the USA carry warnings: '*As in all fluoride toothpastes, keep out of the reach of children under 6 years of age. If you accidentally swallow more than used for brushing, seek professional assistance or contact a poison control center immediately.*'
- Many toothpastes also contain triclosan, which can produce toxic dioxins when in contact with water.
- Formaldehyde can appear under many names, for example methyl aldehyde. It is commonly found in shampoos, nail varnishes and moisturisers. It is banned in Sweden and Japan. In December 2003 it was linked to leukaemia and in January 2004, to lung cancer.
- Talc has a similar formula to asbestos. Baby products warn on the bottle that it should not be breathed; yet it is in many face powders. It has also been linked to ovarian cancer.
- Propylene Glycol is used for skin 'glide'. It is frequently found in moisturisers, face creams and even baby wipes. It is the sister product to commercial anti-freeze. Workers handling it must use protective clothing and gloves, because it burns the skin!

- Dark hair dyes contain paraphenylene diamine, which can cause cancer in rats after exposure to hydrogen peroxide. They also contain ammonia, a basic toxin. A number of neck, head, bladder and kidney cancers have been linked to these dyes.
- Nail varnishes and cleaners often contain xylene, formaldehyde and toluene and are known to cause liver damage and skin and respiratory irritation. Toluene also affects the endocrine system and is an oestrogen mimic. You may be surprised to learn that your nails are actually porous so these chemicals can easily be absorbed by the body.
- Lipstick often contains isopropyl alcohol, which damages DNA, and the colouring can use lead, titanium, zinc or aluminium – the latter being implicated in Alzheimer's. These heavy metals are dangerous if ingested and across a lifetime the average woman is expected to ingest 20 kilos of lipstick!
- Perfume and perfumed products can be a mixture of over 100 different ingredients none of which needs to be named on pack, yet many are endocrine system disrupters.

In 2003 a Royal Commission appointed in the UK, typically by the Queen and the Prime Minister, concluded that there were 4000 ingredients we normally come across in our daily lives, most of which were probably toxic and many probably carcinogenic.

This list includes household cleaners, detergents, polishes, sprays, bleaches and even washing-up liquid.

Some toxins can damage the DNA and the genes. Others may mimic the action of oestrogen, a female hormone, in the body. Is it any surprise then that prostate cancer has now been found to be caused by a substance called DHT, formed when a man's declining levels of testosterone are activated and changed by localised oestrogen (Thompson, Texas 2003)?

Every free-thinking person should look for non-toxic alternative products.

Two of Epstein's prime concerns are that there is no proper regulation of what goes into many of the products you buy for your home and that, even if an ingredient is disclosed on the label, the great majority of people have no idea of its toxicity.

He is also worried about the mix of chemicals you come into

contact with everyday. For example, using two different products on the human face may cause a chemical reaction between some of their ingredients, which subsequently produces a carcinogen.

In case you don't feel that frequent use of SLS making the skin on your hands more permeable is much of a problem, consider this: A recent study showed that the new Euro coin when taped to the back of the hands of members of a research group, resulted in severe irritation and even blistering after 48 hours.

Clearly members of the general public are not going to go around like this in their normal daily lives, but the problem was put down to nickel in the coins. Nickel is believed to be linked to prostate cancer as it can displace the zinc stores in the prostate. Making your skin more porous is not a good idea.

It has been calculated that American men use on average 10 personal care products per day whilst women use 13 personal care and six cosmetic products. Some products like hand soaps are used more than once. This makes the number of possible carcinogenic 'hits' on your body very high, even for babies and young children.

Recent studies have shown that American women can have almost four times the level of toxins in their bloodstreams that American men have, and it has been concluded that this is largely due to their greater usage of cosmetics, toiletries and household products.

In 2003 Professor David Feldman of Stanford University voiced the view that 'the cumulative effect of many of these toxins, which act as oestrogen mimics, may be cumulative'.

Dr Ana Soto of Tufts looked into this, taking ten commonly found toiletry ingredients (each of which was known to mimic the action of oestrogen when in the body) but each at government determined 'safe levels'. In animals, the ten combined to give a full oestrogen response.

There is no safe level for these toxins. You must seek out a supplier of toxin-free products. Epstein's Cancer Prevention Coalition name Neways as such a company and companies using all natural and non-chemical ingredients are springing up everywhere. Find one – you owe it to your body and your immune system.

Q11. What are the main lifestyle factors that increase my risk of cancer?

(i) Alcohol

Alcohol is a chemical poison and has many negative effects, but particularly it overworks the liver potentially causing damage, produces dangerous free radicals, and causes immune system depletion. It is also a neurotoxin damaging the brain and the nervous system. In November 2002, a study linked alcohol consumption with breast cancer in women. Apparently it is thought to stimulate oestrogen production, and a woman's risk of breast cancer increases by 6 per cent for every drink consumed per day (*British Journal of Cancer* vol 87). Alcohol is also implicated in oesophagal, stomach and colon cancer. An occasional glass of Cabernet Sauvignon may have antioxidant benefits. Better to stick to red grape juice. People with cancer should avoid alcohol because it puts stress on an already over-worked liver.

(ii) Tobacco

The packets have health warnings. They are there for a reason. Smoking causes severe free radical release in the body. It is madness to smoke without accepting you are greatly increasing your odds of getting cancer especially after 55 years of age. If you smoke, stop now!

Statistically, even one cigarette a day has the same odds of causing cancer as 20.

Worryingly even non-smokers get smoke-related lung cancer. Cancer Research UK announced findings in autumn 2002 that showed people living with a 20 a day smoker were exposed to six-times the smoke levels of people living in a smoke-free household.

People who work in smoky environments are at risk. Roy Castle's death was attributed to passive smoking; although a non-smoker himself he frequently entertained and played the trumpet in smoke-filled clubs.

The Government should ban smoking in all public places; it is a nonsense to subject children and non-smokers to the selfish whim of a minority of the population.

Women are especially at risk from tobacco smoke. Women have two X-chromosomes in their DNA, men only have one in their DNA. A gene on that X-chromosome causes a carcinogenic factor to appear in the airways of smokers. So women smokers have roughly twice the risk of men who smoke the same number of cigarettes. (Siegfried, University of Pittsburgh). Oestrogen further increases the presence of this factor. Your daughter must not smoke. If they smoke, girls in their sexually formative years, especially those taking the pill as well, increase their risk of breast cancer by a staggering 70 per cent later in life.

(iii) Oestrogen

Men – please do not skip this section, it applies just as much to you as to women.

It used to be the case that 50-year-old men had little oestrogen in their bodies, whilst their 50-year-old wives who had been through the menopause had seen theirs decline by about 40 per cent, just enough to stop them ovulating.

Sadly, this is just no longer true.

Think instead of an 'oestrogen pool' in your body, made up of natural oestrogen, synthetic oestrogen (from products like 'the pill' and HRT) and chemicals that mimic the action of oestrogen (like certain pesticides or ingredients of toiletries and perfumes). Now you start to get the picture.

Oestrogen is known to help spread cancers (NCI, USA). Dr Ana Soto of Tufts showed clearly that the plastic dishes in which she kept her cells, leached oestrogen mimics from the plastic into the cells and proliferated cancer.

Oestrogen: The Killer in Our Midst is a simple book that will tell you much, much more about the dangers of this 'hormone' and what to do if you want to avoid or beat a hormonally driven cancer. There is also a lot of information on our website.

But please be absolutely clear. This 'oestrogen pool' is the driving force in most hormally driven cancers like prostate, melanoma, breast, ovarian and colon. In 2003 Dr Thomson of the University of Texas, Houston, showed oestrogen turns testosterone (which declines in men as they age and is perfectly safe) into nasty DHT. In 2000 researchers in Birmingham showed localised oestrogen was implicated in colon cancer.

In 2002 oestrogen was implicated in melanoma and skin cancers and recent research showed that people who had had skin cancer at some point in their lives went on to get second cancers at a much higher rate than normal. All the second cancers were also oestrogen-driven (**icon** – Cancer Watch).

But, of course, oestrogen is best known for its link to female cancers like breast and ovarian.

An excess of oestrogen can deplete vitamin B levels in the body. Certain B vitamins like folic acid are essential to good cell copying systems. Oestrogen also acts to depress oxygen levels within a cell, which is a condition that encourages a cancer cell to form. Most importantly oestrogen is known to help rogue cancer messages bind to receptor sites on cancer cells, turning them rogue.

Even in small amounts, it is a very powerful immunosuppressant. In excessive amounts, oestrogen is a very powerful and very dangerous hormone in women and men.

Two hundred or more years ago women naturally regulated their oestrogen levels. Their periods started around the age of 16 to 18 and ended age 38 to 40; they had four babies on average and breast-fed them for nine months to two years. Nowadays, changing diets and lifestyles, less babies and breast-feeding has increased the average number of periods a woman has by about 60 per cent or so. Thus the exposure to these oestrogen peaks has also grown significantly.

A Swedish study has linked both late menopause and short menstrual cycles with increased rates of lung cancer.

But it is breast cancer that produces the greatest alarm. The World Health Organisation (WHO) in 1985 linked the oestrogen contraceptive pill to increases in invasive cancers. Nowhere more so than in breast cancer.

To have ever taken the pill increases a woman's chance of breast cancer by 26 per cent; to take it into her 30's increases risk by 58 per cent and in her 40's by 144 per cent. (Cancer Research UK).

HRT creates the same sort of problems. A recent report in the *Lancet* (Vol 360, pages 942-4) concluded that there is a significant increase in the risk of breast cancer, strokes and blood clots on the lungs. HRT was determined to be the actual cause of some breast cancers in women taking it. An eight-year study in the US testing a mixed synthetic oestrogen and progesten pill was stopped in 2002 after only five years as one cancer, breast cancer, had seen a doubling amongst the sample. The oestrogen-only part of the test was allowed to continue and indicated an increased cancer risk at over 27 per cent. Cancer Research UK was adamant in a press release in October 2002 that the risks of HRT outweighed the protective benefits. Cancer Research UK's million women study in 2003 concluded that oestrogen-only HRT caused a 26 per cent increased risk of breast cancer. However, we should have known all this for years. In 1995 the Boston Nurses Study showed the same 26 per cent figure (121,000 women tested for 18 years).

In November, Professor Bruno Muller-Oerlinghausen, Chairman of Germany's Commission on Safety in Medicines, likened HRT to thalidomide in the 1960s!

The problem for women lies in a degree of misinformation. The HRT business – and make no mistake, this is big business, in 2003 there were 2.2 million women in the UK on HRT – is defended by powerful bodies who seek to 'muddy the waters' and hope to convince women that risks are in fact minimal. HRT is often recommended to prevent osteoporosis (usually the result of too much dairy and too little magnesium in our Western diets – see *The Tree of Life: The Anti-Cancer diet* for more information), or hot flushes. However oestrogen levels at menopause fall by 40 per cent, whereas natural progesterone levels fall by almost 100 per cent. It is the sudden imbalance between these two hormones that causes the hot flushes. Natural progesterone supplementation may address the same problem and there is even some indication that it reduces the risks of ovarian cancer by 50 per cent according to Dr Schildkraut at The Duke Cancer Centre, Carolina. (But beware; synthetic progesterone is certainly not beneficial. In research studies it is linked to increased rates of cancer – see our website for more details.)

In both men and women fat stores can produce oestrogen. Overweight women can have higher levels of oestrogen circulating in their bodies after menopause, than thin women had in their prime.

Finally, the new breakthrough breast cancer drugs are called aromatase inhibitors. "What do they do?" Well silly, they aim to cut the high levels of oestrogen circulating in post menopausal women and driving their cancers. "But I thought doctors were prescribing HRT because women had low levels after menopause?!" And so ends another myth.

(iv) A sedentary lifestyle and being overweight

We have already talked about the need to have movement to get the lymph system flowing and reduce pollution around the cells.

We also covered the reasons why overweight people are 40 per cent more likely than the norm to develop a cancer. Remember that the increased risk from smoking is only 25 per cent!

But how do you know if you are in the danger zone?

Most measurements seem too complicated for the normal person. I'm a fully qualified fitness trainer and the Body Mass Index (BMI), which is the official system we are taught to use, is totally meaningless to the average person. It might be helpful to know your fat content and there are simple machines, probably at your local gym, that will tell you. Weight to height is not always strictly relevant because a body builder who puts on muscle may find he weighs more than a slightly fat friend of the same height, simply because muscle weighs more than fat. Bone density also plays a part.

However the charts on the following page give you some clue as to whether or not you are at risk.

I really must caution that these figures are just generally indicative and more individually accurate figures can be made from an estimation of your fat content linked to height and bone structure.

(v) My mother's pregnancy!

There are some dangers you can do little about!

Scientists have analysed 10,000 cases of children's cancer using the British National Registry of Childhood Tumours, and concluded your **mother's age** during her pregnancy makes a lot of difference.

64

Men				
Height	Underweight	Healthy weight	Overweight	Obese
5 ft 1in	below 48	48-63	63-74	74+
5 ft 4in	below 53	53-68	68-80	80+
5 ft 7in	below 59	59-73	73-86	86+
5 ft 10in	below 64	64-79	79-93	93+
6 ft 1in	below 69	69-85	85-103	103+
All weights shown are in kilograms				

Women				
Height	Underweight	Healthy weight	Overweight	Obese
5ft 0in	below 44	44-56	56-67	67+
5ft 3in	below 48	48-60	60-72	72+
5ft 6in	below 53	53-66	66-78	78+
5ft 9in	below 57	57-72	72-85	85+
6ft 0in	below 62	62-79	79-93	93+
All weights shown are in kilograms				

Children with acute lymphoblastic leukaemia, which accounts for a quarter of all childhood cancers were born more often to older mothers.

Mothers aged between 35 and 39 were 30 per cent more likely, and mothers aged 40 and above were 88 per cent more likely than those of 25 to 29 to have a child with this disease.

Unconnected to this, Swedish researchers have shown that three-quarters of 34 **perfumes and perfume toiletry products** tested, contain phthalates (oestrogen mimics) and particularly di-ethylhexyl phthalate. The urine of American women, in a second study, showed the by-products, and at levels many times higher than in corresponding men.

Numerous studies have shown that these phthalates are linked to male reproductive problems in boys born to these women; undescended testicles and testicular cancer being two of them.

Your cancer could have started before you were born.

(vi) Stresses and lifestyle

This area is complex and is tackled in far more detail in section III of this book. For now, here are three examples of the problems that can be caused:

- Stress particularly depletes B vitamins and causes the production of steroids in the body. This has a negative effect on the immune system, the endocrine system and localised cellular biochemistry. All these lead to an increased risk of rogue cell production and a failure by the immune system to cope.
- There has been a study undertaken by SAS (the airline) linking irregular sleeping patterns in long haul stewardesses with depleted levels of melatonin and increased risks of cancer.
- Depression causes physiological changes in the blood count and reduces the blood's oxygen carrying ability. Since cancer cells hate oxygen, depression actually favours cancer. Depression also brings about localised hormonal changes and localised toxin production both of which increase the risk of forming cancer cells.

You need to spend time on your body and your mind.

Q12. What are the main dietary factors that increase my risk of cancer?

The types of cancer that are most affected (positively and negatively) by diet are those which are largely hormone driven (e.g. oesophageal, liver, pancreatic, colon, breast, prostate, stomach). Throughout this book there are frequent mentions of diet so I will not labour the point. The essential discipline is, 'Eat less meat, less animal fat and more vegetables and fruit. Think nourishment; think nutritious.'

(i) Dairy foods

We are the only animals that drink the milk of different species such as cows, goats and sheep. Normal milk contains extra hormones that neither men nor women want like oestrogen, factors that affect your insulin levels, pesticide residues from fields, animal fat and so on. If the cows have been fed growth hormones and antibiotics, traces of those will be found in their milk too.

Professor Jane Plant, who herself had breast cancer, has looked into the effect of dairy products on breast and prostate cancers concluding that there is a direct link. She believes it is an, 'all or none' situation. Even taking in small amounts of dairy (for example, a bar of chocolate, milk in a coffee, even a 'live organic yoghurt') increases the risk of these two cancers. Like smoking, you can't be a non-smoker who still just has one a day.

Scandanavian research in 2000 concluded that 'there is a direct link between consumption of dairy foods and testicular and prostrate cancer rates'.

Another Swedish study (*Am. J. Clin. Nutrition* Nov 2004) concluded that large amounts of dairy increased ovarian cancer risk. Apparently drinking more than a pint a day of milk doubles a woman's risk.

Part of the problem concerns Insulin-like Growth Factor (IGF1) which can throw normal hormone levels out and affect cellular environments negatively whilst increasing oestrogen levels. IGF1 has been shown to pass from the intestines into the bloodstream in mice in small amounts (6 per cent) but this increases to 68 per cent if cassein is present. Cassein is a milk protein. IGF1 has been linked to cancer (NCI).

In another test, even a small amount of butter, or margarine (which often contains dairy products), was found to suppress the body's detoxification enzymes just when you need them (Strang Cancer Prevention Centre, New York).

(ii) Meat, animal fat and farmed fish

Animal fat is a saturated fat. It promotes all manner of cancers and animal fat should be cut to a minimum. It stimulates prostaglandins (see eicosanoids later) in the body which act as inflammatory agents and demand attention from your immune system, thus weakening it. If all this weren't bad enough, meat contains large volumes of the animal's own hormones (which you can reduce by cooking well) and often antibiotics and hormones given to the animal to make it grow bigger and stronger. Farmed fish is not much better, often containing growth hormones, antibiotics and even colourants, like the false pink of smoked salmon. Farmed salmon contains 20 per cent more fat than its wild predecessor.

(iii) Fats and oils in general

By and large fats and oils are bad for you, whatever their source. Any and all fats (even good oils like olive oil) drive up oestrogen levels in the body and increase the risk of hormone based cancers like breast and prostate cancers. Fats also impair the function of white blood cells and thus your immune system. Vegetarians do twice as well as meat eaters in the ability of their immune system to seek and destroy rogue cells. Reducing consumption of fats and oils makes an enormous difference, although of course you must not cut them out completely as they are essential to the normal functioning of the body.

Fats and oils can be classified under three headings:

- **Saturated fats.** These are the worst for you. As with smoking, the end product of eating animal fat or a hydrogenated vegetable oil is a free radical that will cause premature ageing and potentially cancer. This is why you should limit your consumption of red meats and all fried snack foods like crisps,

68

onion rings, peanuts and fast foods, which are invariably covered in this 'killer' fat.

- **Polyunsaturated fats and oils.** A while back these were thought to be the breakthrough and a generation of sunflower oils and margarines purporting to be healthy was launched. They are far better for you than saturated fats and the list includes safflower, sunflower, soybean oil and peanut oil, but they are now believed to be less good for you that was originally claimed.

- **Monounsaturated fats and oils.** Found, for example, in olive oil, walnut oil, flaxseed oil and macadamia nut oil. But beware of some margarines which you think are 100 per cent olive oil. They can contain other fats, oils and even dairy products.

It must be remembered that consuming large amounts of carbohydrate, in excess of your needs, results in increasing your fat stores. Indeed, the Harvard Medical School has just published a rethink of the high carbohydrate, low fat 'idealised' diet decreed by governments 20 years ago. Low carbohydrates, low animal fats, good levels of fruit and vegetables and oils from nuts, seeds and oily fish are some of its features.

(iv) Refined foods and processed foods

White flour is refined and has had almost all of the goodness removed. Look for wholemeal or wholegrain. Don't be misled by brown breads that claim to be 'wheat grain' or 'malted', which is merely refined white flour with added colouring. In malt bread, for example, the malt has dyed the refined white bread brown.

That 'healthy' pasta lunch. Forget it. The chances are the pasta is made from refined, almost worthless flour. Why not adopt my own personal rule? I won't eat a carbohydrate unless it is whole. Nor should you.

All processed foods suffer in the processing. TV dinners and ready-made meals are packages of danger. These foods have to have preservatives to enhance their shelf life, and many are a blend of ingredients and chemicals to achieve an acceptable taste. Undoubtedly, all packaged and processed foods have a collection of E numbers lurking in them. But the biggest problem for all of us is the levels of salt and sugar contained (hidden) in them to enhance taste.

Recent studies in Scandinavia have shown that processed foods such as biscuits, breakfast cereals, crispbreads, crisps and especially overcooked chips contain acrylamides. These are produced when the cooking process exceeds 120°C. Acrylamides are highly toxic.

Many healthy fruit juices are really processed sources of sugar. A famous 'healthy' American natural grape juice declared on the bottle that it contained no vitamin C but it clearly had high levels of sugars. Processing destroys nourishment.

(v) Preservatives

Dried meats, pepperoni, hams, sausages and other processed meats usually contain highly toxic nitrites, especially sodium nitrite. One study in America directly linked hot dog consumption to cancer in children. E numbers are another area for concern and pickling with vinegar is linked to stomach and throat cancers. Smoked meats and fish are not much better.

(vi) Salt, sugar

Both sugar and salt negatively affect your endocrine system. Sugar and refined carbohydrates often consumed in quantity add 'empty' calories to your body (beware foods like pizza and pasta), and encourage insulin production, which in turn can increase oestrogen levels. Fizzy soft drinks can have 10 spoonsful of sugar per can. So called 'healthy' drinks like Ribena can be even higher. Even more worrying is that glucose is the favourite food of the cancer cell. So avoid it at all costs especially if you have a cancer.

Salt is the silent 'killer'. It is estimated that the average American male consumes 12–16 grams per day and in the UK it can be 10 grams. Recently the FSA has said 6 grams for adults and 3 grams for children are the correct targets but in *The Tree of Life: The Anti-Cancer Diet* I argue even these are too high. As animals in the wild we would go days and weeks without salt before finding a salt 'lick'. In Roman times salt was so rare it was used for bartering and as payment (hence the word *salary*). US research in February 2004 suggested 1.5 grams of sodium as a maximum daily level.

As we said earlier, salt poisons your cells and sets up the conditions that breed cancer. Diet therapies like Gerson (see Q25) aim to treat people in part by removing sodium and adding potassium and magnesium back into the diet and cellular structures.

But beware, because most salt and sugar is hidden. Breakfast cereals, a loaf of bread, chicken nuggets and hundreds of processed foods manipulate the salt and sugar content to achieve a more popular taste.

(vii) Caffeine

Caffeine is a poison and is found in soft drinks, coffee, tea and chocolate. It depletes the body of vitamins, especially B vitamins, which are required for healthy cell maintenance and division. It also has a negative effect on the immune system.

(viii) Aspartame?

According to the UK Brain Tumour Foundation, an increase in brain tumours has been noted since aspartame was introduced into the food market in 1981. There is a school of thought, that Aspartame, which is found in a wide variety of diet drinks and yoghurts as the low calorie sweetener, is a neurotoxin and carcinogen. In laboratory tests it has been shown to cause aggressive brain tumours in rats. The arguments continue. Clinical tests are being conducted in the UK specifically looking at links between aspartame and child brain tumours at the moment. Meanwhile there is absolutely no evidence for these claims or rumours where humans are concerned.

(ix) Saccharin

There are a number of US studies with both animals and humans linking saccharin and bladder cancer, although recently another study has suggested otherwise.

(x) Poor diet and poor eating habits

Eating too few vegetables, insufficient fruit, no fibre, too much animal fat, burnt food, fried food, too many chips and crisps, too much sugar and salt, microwaved food; our modern recipe for disaster. Q21 covers this in far more detail.

———————

There are many other possible carcinogens around but as I said at the beginning, this is about reducing the odds. Not smoking, limiting alcohol intake, avoiding fried foods, fats and red meats, dairy and caffeine, the pill, limiting exposure to extreme sunshine and clearing toxic products out of your house would be good and simple places to start and they will give you better odds for avoiding cancer. If you have cancer then they are actions you are strongly and urgently advised to consider.

Q13. What exactly is the immune system?

We have several defence systems in the body which protect us from outside attack. The main one of these is the immune system. A foreign body such as a virus or bacterium entering your body is called an antigen. Viruses and bacteria come in all shapes and sizes and have a complicated coat of protein and fats. Think of them as being like the hundreds of different shaped pieces of a jigsaw puzzle. Each invader of a different illness (e.g. measles or meningitis) has its own specific shape format.

The first thing that happens is that one or two of these invading pieces of jigsaw puzzle are carted off to the 'police station', the local lymph node (for example in your armpits). After a couple of days certain of your white blood cells (called B-lymphocytes) have measured up the invading jigsaw piece exactly and produced a protein coat (or antibody), which can exactly envelop and neutralise it.

Meanwhile the other identical invaders have been multiplying rapidly. The body now makes lots of tailored coats or antibodies to neutralise these. This can take a lot of effort and biochemical reaction, which is why you often have a fever. The masses of neutralised and now harmless cells are then removed by the 'clean up squad' called phagocytes and the liver and kidneys work overtime to break all these dead cells up and clear them from the body via the intestines.

However the B-lymphocytes have to be careful not to start neutralising your own good cells. Your thymus gland produces T-lymphocytes, a pair of which actually tell the B-lymphocytes what to do. They are sort of recognition agents monitoring all things as they pass by in the bloodstream. (As we will see later both melatonin and beta-carotene build T-cell volume in the thymus). They sort out rogue invaders from normal good cells and sound the alert. There are many different formats for T-cells and they are very clever search agents.

But T-cells also work outside the blood stream at the cellular level too. Here they help reject large bacteria, yeasts, outside tissue transplants and cancerous cells. T-cells take quite a while to do their monitoring and rejection job at the cellular level but they are crucial to fighting infection and cancers.

As one example, take the case of a man who had a kidney transplant. He was given immune system supressing drugs to stop rejection of the new transplanted tissue. A while later a routine body X-ray showed he was developing lung cancer, and it was discovered that the transplanted kidney had a very small cancer in it (the lung cancer was thus a secondary). The infected kidney was removed and the T-cells got back to work and neutralised and cleared the lung cancer.

Healthy membranes of B-lymphocytes and T-lymphocytes are crucial to help the locking-on process, fitting the tailored coat over the rogue invader jigsaw piece.

These membranes contain fats which can be oxidised (literally, turned rancid) by free radicals. As we will see later, antioxidants (especially vitamin E) guard them and prevent this from happening, whilst over the last ten years four Nobel Prizes have been won for work on polysaccharides and glycoproteins (See Q 21). These help strengthen the immune system, not just in terms of quantity but in terms of quality too. It is said that in a cancer patient possibly as few as one in a thousand T-cells can actually work efficiently spotting rogue cells. Polysaccharides seem to help clean up cellular membranes and receptor sites to significantly boost the T-cell effect.

Clearly there are things you can do to 'help' your T-cells. But another crucial part of your immune system is your liver and there are lots of things you can do to boost that.

Q14. What has my liver got to do with it?

The liver is the ultimate detoxifier of the whole blood system and hence the whole body. If it is impaired it cannot fully do its job and this creates a 'backlog' throughout the body, leaving toxins in the blood and lymph and other places you do not want them.

All cancer patients suffer from liver inefficiency and overload. The liver may be overwhelmed neutralising the lactic acid produced by the cancer cells, or by processing the toxins already in the body, plus the new toxins from the break down of cancer cells. Dead cells from radiotherapy or chemotherapy will be 'processed' by the liver, as will any intruders like bacteria or viruses. The liver may also be busy tackling the steroids, antibiotics, chemotherapy drugs and pain killers.

The liver contains a large number of bile ducts which, amongst other things, remove toxins from the blood and lymph systems and take them to the colon or intestines. There may well be stones, not a few but literally hundreds the size of grains of sand, clogging up these bile ducts. One estimate quoted that virtually every cancer patient suffered from gallstone blockage in the liver to some degree. Gallstones are caused by cholesterol deposits collecting around clumps of bacteria or pieces of dead parasite and it is not uncommon for cancer patients to have especially 'fatty' livers.

Far worse, the state of the liver can be severely worsened by parasites and by alcohol. As I said before, parasites can take any form, from microscopic ones, to a wide variety of flukes, which particularly inhabit the liver. Cancer patients must not drink alcohol under any circumstances; their liver has enough to do already.

All cancer patients, and people who want to be cancer free, should detox regularly and avoid the consumption of fats during that period. Proprietary detoxes can be purchased in health food stores and benefit the liver, bloodstream and whole body whilst parasite killers can be obtained from good vitamin suppliers. Natural sources of fibre like linseeds and psyllium can be eaten daily, and will also clean your colon as will aloe vera in tablets or liquid form. A clean colon helps you have a cleaner liver.

Choline, inositol, biotin, turmeric, methionine, and milk-thistle

(*Selybum marianum*) all help to 'de-fat' and detox the liver. Herbs are also helpful. Artichoke helps the digestive process and fat breakdown and dandelion helps in fluid absorption.

But to clean it out and de-stone it takes serious effort. There is a detox involving Epsom salts, olive oil, and fresh pink grapefruit that seems to work but lays you low for a couple of days! (Epsom salts is an old-fashioned stomach cleaner and works very rapidly – see Appendix IV for details.) Epsom Salts also provides magnesium, and magnesium is essential for a healthy liver. The French even have bottled waters, advertised as good for your liver because of the magnesium content!

When detoxing the body or the liver it is worth taking ornithine before going to sleep as the detoxification often results in poor sleep patterns.

Every cancer patient should do everything in their power to get their liver back into tip-top working order. Cut the bad fats, animal fats and dairy from your diet; avoid alcohol; detox; introduce herbs that help; try the liver flush and cleanse; and think about an anti-parasite and anti-yeast campaign.

Finally, you may even think about using coffee enemas, which help stimulate the liver and dilate the bile ducts so that as many toxins as possible are cleared out into the intestines. (See Q 24.)

Q15. How can I strengthen my immune system?

The immune system encompasses so many levels. The first line of your defence is probably those friendly bacteria in your gut, whose job it is to 'eat' up yeasts, fungi and microbes when you sleep. Then we have the whole white cell system, your hormones and your liver. But what of your body energy system? So little is known but what is clear from American research is that it 'deserts' an area of your body first – and then you become ill.

Classically people take supplements to boost their immune system. Firstly, a word about the use of supplements in general.

There is a school of thought that says, 'If we all ate properly we wouldn't need supplements'. This, quite simply, is not true.

For example, even if we ate properly we would be very unlikely to get more than 60 IU (International Units) of vitamin E inside us per day whereas 400 IU is a good level for cancer prevention and scientists regularly use levels of 1000 IUs when conducting anti-cancer experiments.

Our soil, and therefore the vegetables grown in it, have been depleted of nutrients over the last 100 years. In February 2004 studies by David Thomas, a minerologist, using the UK Government's own figures showed significant losses in key minerals like calcium, iron, potassium and magnesium in our fruit and vegetables in the years from 1940 to 1990.

This is nothing new. The US Senate concluded (and it is in the records) that laboratory tests prove that US farm soils are depleted as are the fruit, vegetables, nuts, eggs and even milk produced. It also concluded that people were developing mineral deficiencies and this could only be corrected by supplementation. And that was in the Senate minutes in 1936!

Even if you did regiment yourself to the ideal diet could you guarantee to eat it every day in the modern world? Could you get enough omega 3 if you went on a skiing trip, without taking cod liver oil pills, or get enough beta-carotene if you are on a two-day business trip?

As we will see in the coming sections, almost every cancer

patient is both nutritionally deficient *and* nutritionally toxic. And there are several studies that conclusively show that by taking antioxidants, vitamins and minerals you can and will correct this, greatly improving your chances of survival. The detractors – and you will even find these in hospitals – are simply talking rubbish.

The American Cancer Society reported in 2003, on a study running between 1992 and 1997. Over 148,000 people were researched using questionnaires and those who had taken multi-vitamins during the 1980s at least four times per week had 30 per cent less incidence of colon cancer, the cancer studied.

Moreover, the study of vitamins and minerals is still in its infancy. In the last five years alone, vitamin D and vitamin K have been shown to have significant anti-cancer benefits at levels far greater than the Government RDA levels. Vitamin D is only really available to you through the action of sunshine, or via fish oils (a little is obtained via dairy). During winter in Europe, the anti-cancer dose is virtually *only* obtainable via supplementation. Interestingly the Royal Marsden is giving cancer patients vitamin D supplements to help in the treatment programmes!

Who says we are likely to eat properly anyway? The fact is that at least two thirds of the population do not. They like their waffles, crisps, croissants, butter, cheese, coffee, sugar, cakes and steaks. Half of their children never put a red, yellow or green vegetable in their mouths. Having such restricted diets risks people failing to ingest some of the more 'rare' trace elements such as boron, found to be vital in the anti-ageing process.

Virtually all the top anti-ageing experts in the USA take supplements.

You can think of supplements in three ways:

- Insurance: for instance, a quality multivitamin and multi-mineral supplement ensures you ingest the trace elements you need every day
- Top up: for instance, vitamin C is water soluble, as is beta-carotene. They leave the body inside three hours. Athletes lose a lot of vitamins during exercise especially vitamin B. No one eats enough vitamin E. 40 per cent of the population is deficient in magnesium.

- Corrective: for instance, cod liver oil and coenzyme Q10 correct deficiencies in our food patterns, or those arising with age.

Supplements perform a highly useful role within a healthy diet especially when we need to kick-start a health programme. However it must be recognised that they are supposed to 'supplement' and in the longer term you should be restructuring your diet to reduce the dependency upon them as prime sources of vitamins. When you eat a red pepper or a carrot you get so much more than beta-carotene. Apart from other vitamins like vitamin C you get a wealth of supportive carotenoids, cofactors, and bioflavonoids, which are simply not present in a standard vitamin pill. As Liebowitz said, *'food is an important ingredient in a balanced diet'*.

And this is a crucial point. After August 2005 and the new EU regulations (which seem to both defy scientific evidence and logic), you can expect virtually all vitamin supplements in Europe to be synthetic, not natural. Who is to say that these perform anything like as well as the previous natural ones? Certainly in recent press criticisms of vitamin supplements, the accusations invariably concerned synthetic, not natural products.

It is crucial that you try to find supplements sourced naturally (like 'd' vitamin E). Health food companies will increasingly turn to blueberries, spirolina, wheatgrass, raspberries and chlorella as a way of providing vitamins and antioxidants if these loony laws come into effect.

If you are unsure of what supplements you might need you can be tested for vitamin and mineral deficiency.

(i) Vitamin and other supplements

The next four questions and answers specifically address the whole issue of particular supplements, proven scientifically to have a positive effect in the fight against cancer. These sections include information on antioxidants (especially the 'magnificent six' – beta-carotene, vitamin C, vitamin E, selenium, zinc and coenzyme Q 10), vitamins and minerals, herbs and hormones.

(ii) Detoxing

These are ideas to strengthen your immune system:

- Cut out fats, animal fats, dairy and oils from your diet completely for a week or so.
- Take 200 mgs per day of milk-thistle (*Silybum marianum*), to strengthen the liver. It helps it to detoxify itself and actively repairs liver damage.
- Liquid detoxes are simple to buy and use. There are also proprietary herbal detox mixtures available for liver cleansing including lipase, methionine, choline and inositol to help 'de-fat' the liver, plus biotin to help vitamin C work. Other herbal mixtures will help kidney function. The cleaning of the liver and kidneys for three to 10 days is essential after radiotherapy, chemotherapy or for the killing of yeast and parasites. The liver must be restored to full working order.
- Make your own juices and go on a juice diet; natural, freshly prepared juices have a serious fan club. There are plenty of books on the subject (see later).
- Drink copious amounts of water; at least 1.5 litres per day (and up to 3 litres during radiotherapy) this helps expel toxins and relieve the immune system.
- Take adequate fibre; this helps by expelling toxins from the colon after they have passed from the liver. Proprietary fibre brands containing psyllium, pectin (apple fibre), prune powder, flaxseed, Slippery Elm and hosts of other ingredients are easy to buy but must be taken with lots of water. Two tablespoons of linseeds sprinkled on the breakfast cereal are a simple to use source of fibre and omega 3.
- Have vegetarian days; and at least once per day, eat organic complete brown rice and eat two portions of fruit and six to eight of vegetables especially pulses such as lentils and mung beans.

(iii) Yoga, acupuncture, cranial osteopathy and reiki

Acupuncture will balance the body energy systems and natural pulses. It is very powerful and now recognised by the NHS. It works by linking the external aura or energy fields to the internal organs in a much more balanced and strengthening way. Like cranial osteopathy it helps get body energy where it is needed.

Both of these, along with reiki have been proven to measurably increase the strength of the immune system.

Surprisingly (or not, depending upon your beliefs) certain forms of yoga can strengthen your immune system by up to 30 per cent, again probably because they re-energise you, move your lymph system and they are known to expel toxins. New participants in these classes actually smell, as a huge volume of toxins is so quickly removed. All of these energy and immune boosters are covered in more detail later in the book.

Of course, the other way of strengthening your immune system is to cut out the carcinogen suspects listed in the previous answers. For example mobile phones in one study were claimed to reduce the localised immune system around the ear/head area by up to 30 per cent when held to the ear for a prolonged period.

This whole area is discussed more fully in Section III.

Q16. What are the main antioxidants that could help?

In 1986, the US National Cancer Institute conducted a study in rural China amongst 38,000 people. Over a five year period the local population took various antioxidants. One group used the antioxidants beta-carotene, vitamin E and selenium at twice the RDA (which, as we know, is a pretty low figure). Within one to two years after commencing the study, cancer death rates started to fall, and after five years were 13 per cent lower than the control sample. Mortality declined by 21 per cent. This research was published in 1993.

In August 2003 French scientists released the results of their Su. Vi. Max study involving 17,000 men and women aged 35–60. Half received a supplement containing five antioxidants: Vitamins C and E, beta-carotene, zinc and selenium. Across the seven years of the study the risk of men developing cancer fell by 31 per cent and death rates for men and women fell by 37 per cent.

These are but two studies of many, but both show beyond all reasonable doubt that providing nutritional supplements helps both prevent cancer and increase survival time. Did the Government shout about this? Did the health service pass the message on to all of us? Sadly, no. Yet if the figures were replicated in the UK about 30,000 less people would develop cancer each year, and 50,000 less would die from it. Why wasn't a huge fuss made of these results? Certainly every person with a cancer who rings our **icon** offices in the early stages seems to be nutritionally deficient and vitamins, minerals and antioxidants could make a huge difference to their likely survival.

Antioxidants appear to boost the immune system and guard cells from free radical damage. They do this by binding to the sticky free radical's exposed electron and stopping it from attacking important cellular structures. A simple example of antioxidants at work is to take an apple and cut it in half; the air quickly attacks and oxidises the exposed apple, turning it brown. But if you cover one half in fresh lemon juice it will not turn brown. The lemon juice has acted as an antioxidant.

High doses of vitamin E stop cholesterol oxidation and rejuvenate the immune system in people over the age of 60 back almost to the level seen in young people.

There are many antioxidants together with many powerful vitamins and minerals that improve their functioning.

There are also several very clear and successful studies in the USA on the use of antioxidant megadoses to control existing cancers and prevent their recurrence.

Almost all the anti-ageing experts in the USA agree the following list of most beneficial supplements. I call them the 'magnificent six': beta-carotene, vitamin E, zinc, selenium, vitamin C and coenzyme Q 10.

(i) Beta-carotene and vitamin A

Beta-carotene is the precursor of vitamin A (or retinol) in the body. Vitamin A is crucial in the fight against cancer. There is a large volume of evidence providing a direct link between a low vitamin A level in the body and cancer. One such study, reported in 1993, followed 90,000 breast cancer patients in New England. Another, at the Sloan-Kettering Institute, Manhattan, linked supplementation of vitamin A to an 80 per cent remission rate in Leukaemia.

In a recent study, scientists at the Arizona Cancer Center reported that vitamin A reduced lesions in the skin caused by sunburn. And later in life this reduced skin cancer levels.

It is depressing how many health, nutrition and cancer books confuse beta-carotene and vitamin A. Vitamin A cannot be synthesised in the body and must be taken with food as retinol or in its precursor form, beta-carotene. Whilst you can take vitamin A supplements (cod liver oil would be a good source), it is fat soluble and you should limit your dose. This is because excess vitamin A can be highly toxic and can cause your liver to be poisoned in its attempt to clean the excess out of the body. One friend, acting on misguided advice, took cod liver oil and evening primrose oil in large doses throughout a month and ended up turning a yellowish-grey! Far safer to take a little cod liver oil (max 1,000 mgs) whilst providing your body with good volumes of beta-carotene at the same time. The body only makes the amount of vitamin A that it needs from the beta-catotene, which is water-soluble so excess is quickly flushed from the body.

The first link between human cancer and low levels of vitamin A was in 1941 (Abelsetal) with low plasma levels being linked to gastro-intestinal cancers. Since that time there have been studies linking low vitamin A levels with cancers of the breast, prostate, stomach, colon/rectum and upper digestive tract.

If taken in correct doses, beta-carotene is claimed to cut cancer risk by up to 40 per cent. There are literally hundreds of studies on its efficacy in cancer prevention. (The only danger is for smokers where one study in particular showed an increase in tumours by 13 per cent when the sample were smokers who then took beta-carotene.)

Beta-carotene is the orange pigment in carrots, peppers, apricots and pumpkins. You can also find it in sweet potato, chicory, spinach and kale.

It appears to mop up free radicals and block the proliferation of cancer cells.

Normal supplement amounts are 6 mgs, but anti-ageists recommend 10 mgs to 30 mgs (17,000 IU to 50,000 IU) and some take up to 50 mgs themselves. In one study amongst people with colon cancer 30 mgs per day caused cancer inhibition in 44 per cent of users after only two weeks. Dr Simin Meydani at Tufts studied the effects of 50 mg daily doses and showed that the natural immune system killer cells, which fight off cancer, were at much higher levels in the blood than in normal people.

Beta-carotene supplements should be taken with meals as the vitamin needs fat to help its absorption and it should be spread in two or three doses per day as it is easily eliminated from the body.

(ii) Vitamin E

The ultimate free radical buster!

It appears to inhibit the growth of cancer cells at the local level while at the global level protecting the immune system and particularly the B and T-cells.

It is fat-soluble and stops the oxidisation of fats in the membranes of immune cells, brain cells and blood cells (think of it as stopping the membrane fats from turning rancid). Low intake of vitamin E has been linked to stomach cancer in one major Italian research study and to bladder cancer in a study from the MD Anderson Cancer Centre (**icon** – May 2004). It has also been shown to protect against lung cancer caused by pollution.

Vitamin E levels in green vegetables have particularly declined over the last 100 years due to soil depletion. A lettuce now contains one sixth of the vitamin E it had in 1900.

It can be found naturally in soya, nuts, seeds like pumpkin and sunflower, whole grains, whole wheat enriched flour, spinach and eggs. However it is important to note that from natural sources the most you are likely to ingest a day is only about 25–40 IU. Put out a bowl of organic pumpkin, sunflower and sesame seeds to nibble during the day (and throw away the packets of crisps and peanuts using hydrogenated oil).

Inorganic iron destroys vitamin E, while selenium helps it work. In turn, vitamin E helps vitamins A and C work.

About 60 per cent of the daily dose of vitamin E is expelled in the faeces so it needs to be constantly replaced.

Just to make life a little more complicated, there are several forms of vitamin E. Most available in the UK are tocopherol vitamin E's.

However, *America's Life Extension* magazine reported in spring 2002 that tocotrienol vitamin E has been shown to inhibit oestrogen positive receptor sites by as much as 50 per cent. Indeed they recorded that tocotrienol usage could cut tamoxifen requirements for women by 75 per cent. (Tocotrienol vitamin E is not in the EU approved list of medicines and so must be obtained from the USA.)

Tocotrienols seem to collect in breast tissue and keep the tissue soft.

Ideally you should take about 400 IU's of vitamin E per day, although some scientists recommend 1000 IU's. Take it in the '*d*' form (this indicates it is from natural sources) and ideally as a mixture of all four tocotrienols and all four tocopherols (*d-alpha, d-beta, d-delta* and *d-gamma*).

(iii) Selenium

Selenium and vitamin E are synergistic, which means that they work better together than each on their own. Low selenium levels have been linked to cancer both of the stomach and breast. And the UK diet is the lowest in Europe for selenium intake, probably because of our soil, and our low consumption of garlic (garlic contains good levels of selenium). With vitamin E it helps protect against membrane damage; and it acts to replace certain harmful chemicals and heavy metals in the body, for example, mercury. Finally, selenium has an anti-viral and anti-bacterial action freeing up the immune system to fight off cancer.

In parts of China where the soil is rich in selenium, cancer has almost no presence, and there are estimates that a good selenium level in the body reduces cancer risk by 20 per cent.

Selenium is found in lobster, tuna fish, onions, broccoli, tomatoes, wheat germ and bran. Smoking, high intakes of polyunsaturated oils and fats and ingestion of mercury and lead cause a decline in its levels in the body. Fish oils contain quite good levels of selenium.

It is often claimed that eating two to three Brazil nuts per day provides your total requirement. Sadly there is a catch. The nuts must still be in their shells. Unshelled nuts come from a different area with low selenium and, in light, may have started to go rancid and become selenium depleted. But nuts in their shells come from an area quite high in radioactivity. So you just can't win!

Take the supplement but don't overdo it, as it is very powerful and not totally understood. The normal daily dose is 50–100 mcgs but you can go as high as, but not exceed, 200 mcgs.

(iv) Vitamin C

Linus Pauling, the pioneer of vitamin C, felt you should take 3–4 gms per day and up to 10 gms if you were ill. Nowadays there are claims about liver damage, and one study even claimed it caused cancer in excessive amounts, although there seem to be no confirmatory studies or categorical evidence for this. According to one study, women with breast cancer who take at least 10 gms of vitamin C live 16 times longer than those who don't.

Vitamin C seems to help strengthen cell membrane walls in the immune system, weaken cancer cell walls and neutralise aflatoxin (see section on parasites) amongst other more general healing and immune system benefits.

Neil Riordan (Aiden Clinic, Arizona) has published many articles on vitamin C (for example, *British Journal of Cancer* Vol 84, No. 11). He states that in his experience up to 46 per cent of cancer patients have scurvy or a lack of vitamin C.

Vitamin C brings about cell death in cancer cells; large doses cause the build up of hydrogen peroxide in cancer cells. Normal cells contain an enzyme, catalase which breaks this down, but cancer cells do not, resulting in their death. Lymphocytes in healthy people store large amounts of vitamin C ready to attack forming cancer cells.

He has also noted that several nutrients (quercetin, grape seed extract, biotin, vitamin K and lipoic acid) significantly promote the healing effects of vitamin C.

It is always better taken in the ester form as it is better for our stomachs than the straight ascorbic acid form.

Rosehips contain bioflavonoids and certain enzymes, which help assimilate vitamin C into the blood stream. Studies are currently underway on two citrus flavonoids (nobiletin and tangeretin) which substantially influence brain tumour invasion (ie the process of sending out rogue cells into secondary tissue such as the brain).

Vitamin C is water-soluble and passes through the body in about three hours, so it is best taken in smaller amounts at regular intervals or it time release capsules. It is particularly helpful in infection and healing and Dr Pauling actually found it would decrease infections by 25 per cent and cancers by 75 per cent if taken in 1–10 gm doses.

The best natural sources are red peppers, berries, citrus fruits, green vegetables, cauliflower, sweet and normal potatoes and tomatoes.

When taking large amounts you should take magnesium to avoid kidney stones.

(v) Zinc

It is arguable that zinc per se is not an antioxidant but helps others do their job. It particularly helps the action of vitamin C and it works better itself when combined with vitamin A.

Zinc is credited with a vast number of things, from accelerating healing time to slowing the greying of hair and preventing white spots on fingernails. Zinc is very important for a healthy prostate gland and it is crucial in wound healing.

Alcoholics and people taking B-6 need higher amounts of zinc. It is found in meat, eggs, pumpkin seeds, sesame seeds, sunflower seeds and wheat germ and brewers yeast, shellfish and oysters.

Available as zinc sulphate or gluconate, 15–300 mgs can be taken, although recommended levels are 15–50 mgs.

Ingesting cow's milk and dairy products blocks the absorption of zinc. In children especially this depletes appetites and makes for 'picky eaters' so it is wrong to give milk to young children who do not eat a wide and varied diet on the basis that at least it is giving them nourishment. It actually prevents them from being nourished by restricting their appetites.

(vi) Coenzyme Q10 (CoQ10)

CoQ10 is a powerful antioxidant that, like vitamin E, protects the fats in membranes from being oxidised by free radicals. It helps stabilise all membranes.

CoQ10 also works inside the energy powerhouse (the mitochondria) in each and every cell in your body. Without it, exhaustion would set in and the immune system would collapse.

It is particlarly important as cancer cells have mitochondria that work abnormally, being unable to metabolise oxygen and producing energy only through a process called glycolysis. CoQ10 may well protect mitochondria from becoming abnormal.

In older people whose immune systems naturally decline with age, 60 mgs per day of CoQ10 produced antibody levels reaching those of young people. Statins, which are being widely distributed to people with heart and cholesterol problems, have been shown to deplete CoQ10 levels in the body and a paper is with the FDA in the USA at the moment.

CoQ10 can cross into the brain and is proven to prevent brain cell deterioration. Recent studies have shown an important role in prevention of dementia, and it can play an important role in patients with brain tumours.

It takes time to work, usually two to three months, and the normal dose is 30 mgs, although people with signs of chronic disease can take more. Studies show that the maximum level in the blood peaks with doses of 100 mgs. Like hormone supplementation, it should not be given to people under the age of 20 who should be producing more than enough anyway.

There are literally hundreds of antioxidants. Antioxidants abound in herbs and plants and many fruits and vegetables whilst some of the 'magnificent six' have many more bioflavonoids and cofactors that help their action. The more antioxidants you consume and the more diverse their source the more protected you are. Here are some others worth exploring:

(vii) Lycopene

Lycopene is another antioxidant found in yellow and orange vegetables, mostly tomatoes, strawberries, peppers, carrots and peaches. The daily dose recommended is about 5–10 mgs. It is part of a package recommended to support a healthy prostate. The other effective ingredients are saw palmetto berries (oil) 150–400 mgs; Korean (panax) ginseng 3–5 mgs; pygeum bark (*Pygeum africans*) 1.5–2.0 mgs; zinc 15 mgs.

Prostate cancer is less common in vegetarians and in Asia where people eat more soya, vegetables, rice and less animal fats and dairy. Lycopene actually binds to fats and lipids in the blood stream helping us overcome our Western diet. A Harvard study showed people with 10 plus servings of lycopene vegetables/fruits per week had 45 per cent less risk of cancer. In particular cooked tomatoes seem to release their lycopene more readily.

(viii) Lemon grass, kaffir lime and watercress

The Thais have more than their fair share of toxins around them but low, low cancer rates. Lemon grass, one of their natural and constant cooking herbs, is supposedly 100 times stronger then beta-carotene as an antioxidant, galanga and kaffir lime leaves are three to five times stronger. Back in the UK watercress, beetroot and a number of natural fresh organic herbs also help boost the immune system more than most vitamin pills.

(ix) Circuminoids

These are phytochemical phenol products that have broad and powerful antioxidant benefits and act both to bind to free radicals and prevent their formation in the first place. They are also known to stimulate glutathione action in detoxifying cells. They work particularly well in conjunction with vitamin E and are found as the yellow pigment of turmeric. Curcumin causes cell death in melanoma cells and several types of cancer cells in laboratory tests.

(x) Grape seed extract and pine bark

Both these substances contain OPCs (oligomeric proanthocyanidins), although they each contain slightly different cofactors. OPCs are very powerful antioxidants, reputedly 20–50 times more powerful than vitamins E and C. OPCs prevent the oxidation process that forms free radicals at the cellular level, and scavenge free radicals throughout the body. Their power as an anti-cancer agent is being researched currently.

Taking antioxidants with chemo and radiotherapy

A question that often crops up is, "Should I take antioxidants whilst having chemotherapy or radiotherapy?" Doctors are divided over this, some saying the antioxidants will neutralise the free radicals from the two treatments that are provided deliberately and specifically to attack the DNA of the cancer cells.

A couple of points are worth considering:

Rarely, if ever, do the same people tell you not to eat carrots, red peppers, apples, brazil nuts, garlic, salmon or oysters, which is rather odd if these antioxidants are so worrying. It is also quite nonsense to suggest that somehow there is a neutralising effect in the blood stream. The biochemistry just doesn't work like that.

John Boik, of the MD Anderson Cancer Institute, Texas, in his excellent reference book *Natural Compounds in Cancer Therapy* produces evidence and references that many antioxidants actually enhance the effect of chemotherapy and radiotherapy.

Recent research (**icon** – Cancer Watch) from the USA clearly argued that healthy cells limited their uptake of antioxidants and would thus protect themselves fully, whilst cancer cells had no such control mechanism and so taking antioxidants was more likely to destroy them. New chemotherapies are also much more selective (e.g. aromatase inhibitors) and do not work as free radicals anyway, so there is absolutely no reason not to take your antioxidants. But do tell your doctor as always, and if there is any dispute, suggest he reads the Boik book – it has over 4000 scientific references and concludes that supplements such as antioxidants really do help get better results from orthodox treatments like chemotherapy and radiotherapy!

Q17. What other supplements might help?

(i) Multivitamin and mineral supplements.

Almost all the top anti-ageing experts in the USA take a good multivitamin and mineral supplement daily. There are some questions over the benefit of iron (and actually quite a lot of concern) and problems with its absorption. Look for supplements that are iron free, or contain organic iron. However the real benefit is in trace but important minerals like boron, magnesium, calcium, phosphorus and manganese. Multivitamins tend to provide poor levels of beta-carotene, vitamins C and E although good levels of certain B vitamins.

One of the biggest problems with all multivitamin and mineral pill supplements is the poor absorption rates; such a pill must dissolve within 30 minutes of hitting the stomach or it will pass through the body without being absorbed. The problem is caused because these multi-pills have the ingredients 'glued' together. It is estimated that up to 85 per cent of multivitamin pills can pass straight through you. Look for colloidal supplements, which are more readily absorbed. The problem of absorption is further worsened for vitamins such as C and beta-carotene, which can be flushed out of the body in less than three hours, as they are water-soluble. There is some debate as to whether any of the C or beta-carotene even reaches the more distant cells of your body. It is better to take small doses of these vitamins frequently in an attempt to keep your cellular system topped up.

(ii) B vitamins

B complex often contains a number of individual B vitamins, which are potent when mixed together rather than used separately. Beware though, that some B complex are yeast based pills and you would be wise to avoid these.

Cooking particularly destroys B vitamins, as does alcohol, caffeine, food processing, the pill (oestrogen) and smoking. A lot of athletes have B deficiency because it is expelled in sweat, being water-soluble

B vitamins particularly help in the nervous system and with cell growth, memory and red blood cell production. B-1, B-2, B-6, and B-12 are essential to the body, whilst low levels of B-2, B-3 and especially B-12 have been linked to cancer. All of these may be found in multivitamin or B complex supplements. But there are others, which are important to consider but not always found in these forms. These are:

- Biotin – essential for vitamin C to work. Good sources are nuts, egg yolk (but egg white destroys it), organic complete rice, fruits and milk. Take 0.3 mgs per day especially if you are on antibiotics.
- Folic acid – critical for the accurate replication of DNA, your genetic code, every time cells divide. It is found in green leafy vegetables, egg yolk, liver, pumpkin, apricots, avocado, carrots and beans and whole grain flour. For cancer prevention, take 400 mcgs per day (never more than 800 mcgs). It is essential at the very point of cancer formation because when DNA divides, mutations can occur and folic acid reduces the risk. It is also crucial for cancer sufferers during radiotherapy treatment. Folic acid helps reduce the risk of colon cancer and is also important in retaining memory as you age.
- Inositol and choline – two separate B vitamins, but they work together. They are crucial for healthy membranes, the immune system (where they aid the work of vitamin E), and they are two of the few substances to cross the blood brain barrier and go into brain cells aiding memory. (Choline is now thought to help stave off Alzheimer's.) Enemies are alcohol, the pill and caffeine.

  The best natural sources are liver, beans, egg yolks, offal, wheat germ and cabbage. But soya lecithin provides both. Daily doses are inositol 250–500 mgs, choline 500–1000 mgs. Take soya lecithin (from soya beans) in capsules (up to 3 gms per day, maximum) or in powder sprinkled over your breakfast cereal. Inositol and choline help keep the liver from being clogged up with fats and thus are very effective in this area of the immune system.
- Vitamin B-12 is involved in over 300 'reactions' in the body. Its full name is cyanocobalmin. It is stored in the liver and shortages of it are not noticed until too late. Unfortunately 73 per

cent of vegetarians have low levels of this essential vitamin, and increasingly the over-50s have shortages too. The best sources are usually quoted as animal, especially offal, but in fact natural chlorella is an excellent source too. Women with breast cancer have lowered levels (Choi, Sang-Woon). It is also deficient in people with Helicobacter pylori and they have more incidence of stomach and gastric cancers.

- B-17 (laetrile or amygdalin) – B-17 or amygdalin is a naturally occurring vitamin identified in 1955 by Ernst Krebs and claimed to be extremely effective in the treatment of cancer or simply in prevention. Its use is controversial because the Federal Drug Administration (FDA) in the USA has not approved it (although why they officially needed to approve a naturally occurring vitamin in the first place is a mystery in itself). A Senate committee (often accused of being biased and with rumoured drug industry connections) seemed unimpressed by evidence that:
  - Three quarters of 80 cancer test patients had seen their cancer tumours go or reduce in size
  - Populations where B-17 is naturally consumed are cancer free (e.g. Hunzaland/Nepal. Mind you, they probably don't have too many mobile phones, processed foods and pesticides in Nepal either!)

The argument runs that 100 years ago we naturally ate far more B-17. It can be found naturally in apricot kernels, apple seeds and peach kernels where it can reach the 3 per cent level, plus the seeds of prunes, plums and cherries, and in walnuts, brazils, cashews, macadamia nuts, millet, buckwheat and cranberries and cranberry juice. The higher the level of B-17 in the kernels the more bitter their taste.

The controversy centres on the fact that the B-17 molecule 'contains' cyanide and is thus dangerous. But then, so does vitamin B-12 and no one complains about that!

Also it is a vast over-simplification. As we said in Q4 the power stations, or mitochondria, are different in cancer cells. They don't use oxygen but burn their fuel, glucose, using an enzyme called glucosidase.

This enzyme converts B-17 into benzaldehyde (an analgesic) and hydrogen cyanide (a poison), thus killing the cell.

Normal cells produce energy using oxygen and an enzyme rhodinase. Rhodinase neutralises B-17.

To put this in context a cancer cell has 3,000 times the glucosidase of a normal cell ensuring that, inside those cells, benzaldehyde and hydrogen cyanide are made in dangerous quantities. So B-17 is like a natural 'search and destroy' homing device for cancer cells.

Clinics using B-17 treatments (along with vitamin megadoses) have been forced out of America across the border into Mexico. It is illegal in California, for example, to recommend any cancer treatment other than surgery, radiotherapy, and chemotherapy. This furthers their dangerous quack image, casting a shadow over the vitamin and stopping proper research. Conversely, disciples of B-17 claim that the pharmaceutical companies are trying to protect the huge profits they make by restricting treatments to ineffective but profitable chemotherapy drugs. Impasse.

Critics were thus horrified in the UK when the Health Authorities banned the prescribing of B-17 in June 2004. Interestingly this occurred the same week that the Government unveiled its new Health Initiative with the theme: More Choice!!

According to *Nutrition Almanac* in the USA five to 35 apricot kernels eaten throughout the day can be a sufficient preventative amount; but people are advised never to eat more than five at one time. Krebs himself recommended taking 10 seeds per day for life.

Tablets or vitamin pills can be obtained and two to four tablets each of 100 mgs is the suggested daily preventative amount. Treatment clinics for cancer patients use both apricot kernels and doses of four to six 500 mgs tablets per day. Tests show cumulative amounts of around 3 gms can be digested safely but it is recommended that no more than 1 gm is taken at any one time.

Great care has to be taken with people undergoing B-17 treatment or metabolic therapy treatment. The by-products of B-17 breakdown and its action will pass to the liver where they in turn are rendered harmless by an enzyme, glucuronide. However, firstly, everybody's levels of this enzyme are different and, secondly, in cancer patients the liver function is likely to be impaired and levels of this enzyme might be low and insufficient to deal with the B-17 action.

B-17 action is supported and enhanced by two protein digestive enzymes; one from pineapple (bromelain), one from papaya (papain).

The two enzymes help to de-mask the outer shield of the malignant cell and although the two enzymes can be taken in pill form it is probably better to eat a pineapple and two papayas, if you can manage it every day!

B-17 is also enhanced in its action by taking 5–6 gms of vitamin C, plus vitamins E and A. Successes with B-17 have involved all these supplements and some critics claim it is these 'extras' that are the real successes.

In Canada, Italy, Mexico, Belgium and the USA oncologists in clinics are currently using B-17 as part of 'dynamic metabolic therapy' and they claim to have good success rates, although there are a few cast iron statistical studies with humans. But on 25 August 2000, the USA FDA and Department of Justice instructed two companies selling the synthetic form of the vitamin, laetrile, to stop supplying it beyond their individual state borders, effectively shutting down their businesses. According to the FDA the status of laetrile is, 'no different than that of any other unapproved drug.'

The curious thing is that this ban extended to the supply of apricot kernels as well! You can, of course, buy apricots anywhere and crack the kernels open yourself and B-17 is available in certain European countries and supposedly even on the German NHS, although I haven't personally checked this.

The US Government has now also banned the planting of bitter almond trees, so they seem unequivocal in their pursuit of B-17. All this from a government that allows melatonin and other hormones to be freely sold in their supermarkets.

Dr Contreras of the Oasis of Hope says that B-17 metabolic therapy is ineffective with cancers of the brain, liver and sarcomas. He should know, as his treatment programmes use it extensively. Supplies of B-17 may still be obtained from the Oasis of Hope.

(iii) Calcium and vitamin D

Low calcium causes a hormone calcitrol to be produced, which enhances fat storage and fat stores more toxins, as I covered earlier. Hence it is important in cancer prevention. Some studies have shown that depleted levels of calcium are linked to breast and colon cancers.

Although the majority of us get more than enough calcium without eating dairy products, talk of brittle bones later on in life has focused more attention on it. In fact the issue with calcium is not intake levels but storage and loss levels from the body. It is easily absorbed, stored and highly reusable as long as vitamin D (particularly D-3) and magnesium are plentiful. Resistance training will cause more of it to be taken into the bones and improve density. But smoking, oestrogen and alcohol, for example, deplete stores significantly.

Controversially, milk and dairy products, the very foods that give Western populations their high blood calcium levels, simultaneously give us our low bone calcium levels. Dairy products, apart from containing hormones, pesticides, and trace metals, block the body's ability to absorb zinc and iron and this in turn greatly imbalances magnesium levels affecting our ability to take the calcium from the blood and bind it into the bones. Osteoporosis usually requires magnesium supplementation and certainly not more dairy consumption. Coral calcium and coral kelp are good non-dairy sources of calcium, magnesium and a host of other minerals. They are currently favoured as cancer fighting supplements in the alternative field as they have an alkalising effect and so help to balance the body's pH. Since both are natural products they have all their minerals in an organic and bioavailable form.

Vitamin D itself has a strong anti-cancer role even though it is only present in small quantities in our food. It significantly affects the incidence of prostate cancer, and the Royal Marsden recommend that breast cancer patients take it. Professor Michael Hollick of the Boston School of Medicine has argued that 25 per cent of the women who die of breast cancer would have avoided the problem if they had taken adequate levels of vitamin D in their lives.

In May 2003 at the Howard Hughes Medical School, vitamin D was shown to reduce colon cancer risk and pre-cancerous polyps in the colon.

Vitamin D has been shown to inhibit the growth of the new blood vessels required to allow a tumour to grow, and it has also been shown to switch stem cells over into normal cells.

Vitamin D can be synthesised by the action of sunlight on our skins. Although the official safety limit is set at 2000 IUs, you can make 10,000 daily in the sun. Sadly black-skinned people cannot make vitamin D this way due to their skin pigmentation. Black people have higher rates of prostate cancer.

A little vitamin D is actually found in dairy but the best source is fish oils.

The RDA is minute at 5–10 micrograms per day and is based on work over 50 years ago. At least five times this level is needed for cancer prevention (Veith).

Vitamin D is important to the growth and maturation of your immune system's defence cells, and Hollick is clear it reduces the risk of about 15 cancers from prostate to ovarian.

(iv) Vitamin K

This is a newcomer into the world of anti-cancer vitamins. The vitamin is found in green leaf vegetables, spinach and broccoli. Recent research has shed completely new information on this vitamin and it has been proven useful in various cancers including liver, colon, stomach, leukaemia, lung and breast.

However the findings required levels higher than you could normally consume so supplementation is essential.

(v) Ellagic acid

Research in the USA has shown that ellagic acid can be helpful in cervical cancers and even stop HPV infection. The method? Patients in the study were given half a cup of raspberries!

Q18. What hormone supplements might help?

Hormones are very, very potent chemicals and, under normal healthy conditions, they are in complete balance in your body. This is called homeostasis. However, it is easy to throw that balance out by eating or drinking 'sugar', by stress, lack of sleep or by absorption of outside hormones. Those that you take in from outside sources tend to be pretty dangerous; those that you make yourself are crucial. A couple of them in particular are powerful cleansers or neutralisers of free radicals in your body. Although none in the UK is available as a supplement except on prescription, many are available at health food and vitamin stores in the USA. Extreme caution is recommended before taking any of them and a conversation with a knowledgeable doctor is essential.

(i) Melatonin

Melatonin is primarily produced in the pineal gland deep inside the brain. However, recently it has also been found produced in the gut and retina. In the pineal it is produced when we sleep and it is directly linked to how well we sleep. The peak of production is usually about one to two hours after falling asleep and it pushes you into a deeper level of sleep. However, levels of production decline markedly as we age to almost nil at the age of 70. (This explains in part why older people sleep less well.) Sleeping with the light on disrupts melatonin production, as does long-haul flying and night shift work. A recent study shows that women who work night shifts have a higher breast cancer rate and it is thought that this is due to their lowered levels of melatonin.

It is made from an essential (ie. one we can't make ourselves and have to eat) amino acid called tryptophan, which is first converted to seratonin, a brain chemical associated with mood, and then to melatonin.

Melatonin is very powerful and acts as a suppressor of oestrogen levels, and also as an antioxidant against free radicals. It is thought to be the only antioxidant capable of entering every cell in the body and potentially neutralising all free radicals. One of the key glands it stimulates is the thymus, which plays a core role in the immune system, being the store of T-cells. The thymus degenerates by 90 per cent as we get older, reducing dramatically the potency of our immune system. In tests with cancer patients 10 mgs of melatonin per night produced a marked improvement in immune systems, in particular improving levels of interferon-gamma, T-cells and interleukin-2, which is a hormone that aids T-cell production.

Breast cancer patients have low levels of melatonin and melatonin use has been found to have a positive effect with breast, prostate and lung cancer. It seems to work best with solid tumours rather than metastasised ones, or those in brain or liver. Normal doses are 3–10 mgs. Some treatments go to 40 mgs although there are dangers of hallucination above 10 mgs. Because it is so powerful it should not be taken for long periods. Melatonin is naturally produced in good quantities until puberty and it should never be given to children. You cannot buy it in the UK, and it is available only on prescription.

(ii) Human growth hormone (Hgh)

Human growth hormone, or somatotropin, is a simple protein produced by the pituitary gland. It is also produced during sleep and again is found primarily in children pre-puberty. It passes into the bloodstream to the liver where it is converted to growth factors DGF 1 and 2, which carry the message to other parts of the body.

Its primary function is to help bones grow and to assist in the transport and utilisation of amino acids, the components of protein. In tests using injections of Hgh with adults, the hormone was shown to reduce fatty tissue and promote lean muscle mass.

It does seem to play an anti-cancer role but this is imprecise and certainly injections of Hgh in adults are not without side effects. Like melatonin, Hgh production falls dramatically with age. Its action seems to be that it is essential to the immune system by producing superoxide radicals. These activate the macrophages that seek and destroy infecting rogue cells. Melatonin itself may increase Hgh levels.

The amino acid argenine has been shown to stimulate the

pituitary to produce Hgh, as has ornithine and, indirectly, choline.

Taking these three supplements has been recommended for increasing Hgh production. The other effective stimulator appears to be exercise, and particularly resistance training, where muscles are deliberately fatigued by heavier than normal weights. Lower body workouts are particularly effective.

Finally, a calorie-restricted diet also produces higher than normal levels of Hgh.

(iii) DHEA (Dehydroepiandrosterone)

DHEA requires healthy kidneys (and adrenal glands) for its production. It particularly helps the immune system to recognise infecting bacteria, viruses and cancer cells. It seems to stimulate T-cell and IL-2 production by protecting the thymus from decline.

It is one of the most abundant hormones in our bodies when we are younger but, again, levels lower significantly as we age and the adrenal glands get smaller.

It is widely believed that a person's risk of cancer may be correlated with the levels of DHEA in the blood or urine. However, to date, opinions are mixed and there is even a little evidence that taking DHEA may promote some cancers causing an increased risk of, for example, prostate or breast tumours. Conversely, several recent studies do show its importance overall in the anti-cancer fight.

DHEA replacement therapy is available in the USA and although people do take it, it really seems to be an imprecise science at the moment. You cannot buy the tablets in the UK, only in the USA.

One suggestion I came across was to take a DHEA precursor, which is found in wild yam, as this would at least allow the body some control over the DHEA levels subsequently produced. (Wild yam, primarily found in China and Japan, is reported to help boost the immune system and overall health.)

Q19. Are there any other important hormones that play an anti-cancer role?

Yes, eicosanoids

Many people, including doctors, have never heard of eicosanoids, although they may have heard of one of their subgroups, prostaglandins. In fact, although eicosanoids have been the subject of Nobel Prizes (Sir John Vane, in 1982), they have been widely ignored.

Eicosanoids are hormones; very, very powerful ones, produced by each and every one of your cells, not by endocrine glands. There are over 100 of them. Because they do not need to travel round the body they don't last long, working and self-destructing in a matter of seconds. This makes analysing them very difficult. Basically they react to the messages provided by the hormones, toxins and nutrients in the fluid around the cell and then activate receptor sites on the surface of the cell to tell it what to do. Some are good and work to protect the cell, some are bad and make matters worse.

What is interesting about them is that you can influence whether you make more good ones or bad ones. Although there are a number of influencing factors, the three most relevant to this book are:

- Consumption of EPA, e.g. in fish oils
- Levels of insulin in the body
- Levels of stress hormones.

Fish oils

Grandma's favourite, cod liver oil, really does work. Indeed, oily fish are a very rich source of a substance called EPA, which is an example of a long-chained omega 3 fatty acid. This has a profound protective effect on the body in many areas. (Some seed oils contain omega 3, however these are short chained omega 3 fatty acids and seem to have a neutral effect in the body.)

Much has been written about 'good' omega 3 fatty acids and

'bad' omega 6 fatty acids. Long ago when we hunted from our caves they were probably in the ratio of one to one in our bodies and even 100 years ago they were one to two. Now the average New Yorker has a ratio of one to 25 (good to bad)

EPA and GLA (a substance from evening primrose or borage oil) are converted into stores of DGLA. But, unfortunately, even nasty old hydrogenated oils can raise the DGLA levels in the body.

The problem comes because DGLA can be used to make any one of the 100 or so eicosanoids, good or bad. And what determines the production of bad eicosanoids is the activity of just one enzyme. Crucially, DGLA is converted by this enzyme into arachidonic acid, which in turn makes only bad eicosanoids such as excess prostaglandins.

Long chain EPA from fish oil blocks this enzyme thus ensuring the balance shifts away from bad towards good eicosanoid production. Only EPA can block this enzyme; evening primrose oil and borage or hydrogenated fats cannot.

All 60 trillion of your body's cells can and do make eicosanoids, so clearly the preponderance of good guys to bad guys is crucial. Those people who take evening primrose oil (e.g. for period pains), should be careful and think seriously about taking a fish oil supplement as well. But remember, because fish oils are high in vitamin A, which has a toxic effect on the liver if taken in excess, you should limit your supplement to 1,000 mgs per day.

Levels of insulin in the body

Insulin stimulates the enzyme that makes bad eicosanoids. This has implications for overweight people, who often flood their bodies with carbohydrates and sugars and thus stimulate excess insulin production.

Levels of stress hormones

Cortisol and steroids, for example, are also known to have a stimulating effect on this same enzyme. Both are produced by the endocrine glands in response to stimuli from the brain. So eicosanoids are the final link in the chain between brain moods and your cellular biochemistry. Negative thoughts, stress and guilt are all factors that switch on bad eicosanoid production through this link with the endocrine system, bathing the localised cellular system in a negative environment.

Other factors

Other substances referred to elsewhere in this book are linked to eicosanoids and their action. Ginger contains sequiterpenes, which inhibit the production of bad eicosanoids (especially prostaglandins and leukotrienes).

In garlic there is a substance called ajoene which limits bad eicosanoid responses and, in turn, has been shown to reduce blood pressure, inflammation, and inhibit cancers.

The original eicosanoid research 20 years ago studied the effect of aspirin (salicylate) in blocking bad eicosanoid production. The Mayo clinic has confirmed this research and showed how just 81 mgs of aspirin per day could reduce cancer risks. They also reconfirmed the effectiveness of omega 3. Hardly a month seems to pass without yet another claim that aspirin helps prevent/beat a cancer. Breast, prostate and colon were all reviewed in research in 2004. Apart from its effect with bad eicosanoids, aspirin helps reduce inflammation and many cancers seem to go through a preliminary inflammation stage before taking hold. Certainly aspirin seems to limit the growth of pre-cancerous intestinal polyps preventing reoccurance of colon cancer. If you do not want to take aspirin, you can always take a morning dose of Aloe Vera which contains salicylate and other similar compounds.

So although this work still needs the finishing touches, there is already strong evidence that eicosanoids have a critical bearing on cellular biochemistry and thus on the cancer potential there.

It cannot be stressed enough that hormones are very, very powerful. Powerful enough to 'trump' anything else in and around the cell.

Q20. What natural herbal or plant supplements might help?

Herbs have been used to treat ailments for thousands of years. The rose gardens surrounding Hampton Court Palace were in fact herb gardens in the middle ages, whilst red clover blossoms were a herb of choice for Hippocrates. Sadly, the 'get-well-quick' mentality of recent decades has seen many long established herbs with proven track records dropped in favour of, for example, antibiotics. Worse, some mischievous elves then tell patients not to take the herbs because they interfere with the drugs! Obviously there are 'contra-indications' in some cases and you should always discuss all herb taking with your doctor, but also ask for the evidence rather than accept sometimes sweeping and factually inaccurate negative statements.

When it comes to cancer treatments, modern medicine contains a huge paradox, especially for the cancer sufferer. Namely at the very moment one needs one's immune system in tip-top order, many of the medical profession's cancer treatments are in fact weakening or destroying it. Sometimes Biological Response Modifiers (BRMs) are given to patients along with the chemotherapy drugs to reduce the side effects and damage to the immune system.

Some natural supplements can have the same desired effect, reducing the damage to the sufferer's immune system or, in the case of the non-sufferer, boosting the whole immune response and actually increasing the odds that this person will not become a cancer sufferer in the first place.

Two common BRMs are often given with cancer treatments. These are hormone-like products called cytokines:

- Interleukins, that stimulate the production of white blood cells
- Interferons, that help the body produce antiviral chemicals and stimulate the destruction of foreign bodies(by stimulating macrophage production).

Much interest in the medical laboratories now centres on natural herbal cytokines, which seem to produce strong immune responses without the side effects.

Whether or not you have cancer the herbal supplements you might consider using are:

(i) Astragalus

Astragalus (*Astragalus membranaceous*) has been around in Chinese medicine for two thousand years. It is known as haung qi, or chi, because it was thought to boost natural body energy and is taken from the root of a plant needing four to seven years to mature. This herb has been used as an immune system booster and specifically to treat burns, abscesses, and for hepatitis. In Chinese hospitals it is now used to help people recover from the negative effects of radiotherapy and chemotherapy.

Its wide usage in China, because it offers a direct boost to the immune system, has been supported by recent tests in the US and has led the medical profession to conclude it does have benefits in the fight against cancer. It is soon to be granted FDA approval as an anti-cancer agent. In tests at the Hiroshima School of Medicine in Japan, it was shown to directly increase B-lymphocyte growth, T-cell, interlukin and antibody production. It seems to have the added benefit of improving the effectiveness of radiotherapy by boosting the cancer fighting system.

Researchers in the USA reported that cancer patients undergoing radiotherapy had twice the survival rates if they took astragalus, and all of the above has been confirmed by the University of Texas. Indeed the University of Texas has conducted extensive research on this herb and given it a glowing report in its actions against cancer.

Astragalus appears to contain bioflavonoids, choline and a polysaccharide, astragalan B. The latter controls bacterial infection and viruses by binding to their outer membranes and weakening them. It is also an important adjunct now in the fight against AIDS.

It should be taken with meals, three times per day with a total intake of around 2,000–3,000 mgs per day.

(ii) Garlic

Garlic (*Allium sativum*) is anti-bacterial and anti-viral, it actively boosts the immune system and people who eat garlic contract less cancers. People who eat garlic more than once per week have half the rate of colon cancer in a study of 42,000 older women in Iowa. And prostate cells exposed to the garlic chemical SAMC grow at only 25 per cent the normal rate. Garlic has been shown to inhibit cancer in all tissues including breast, liver and colon. It should be eaten crushed or raw because cooking destroys its active ingredients. (Take out the green centre and ideally buy it fresh when it is not made up of obvious concentric leaves, and your breath won't smell!)

Garlic is probably most talked about for its ingredient allicin, which actually prevents cancer cell proliferation. Together with other natural flavones it seems to help the immune system by its third party work, like lowering blood pressure and cholesterol levels, whilst exhibiting antiviral and antibacterial activities (e.g. in helping cut yeast and mould infections in the body). Garlic contains good levels of tryptophan, the precursor of seratonin, which is the precursor of melatonin.

Few people mention its selenium and germamium contents, when both are such good strengthening agents in the fight against cancer. They mop up free radicals and, along with the S-ally cysteine and dialyl-sulphide also found in garlic, they neutralise carcinogens. Germamium appears to help transport oxygen into cancer cells. Cancer cells hate oxygen: they cannot metabolise it and so they die. It also helps the body produce higher levels of interferon, a powerful anti-cancer force.

Garlic's action with moulds and yeast also extends to its abilities to neutralise aflatoxins, which they and parasites produce. Research (Soni KB 1997) has shown that garlic enhances a liver enzyme that helps to detoxify aflatoxins before they cause damage.

Garlic also seems to have an effect in protecting the body against the side effects of radiotherapy, particularly from DNA and chromosome damage. Finally, doses of garlic seem to directly inhibit bladder and stomach cancer tumour growth

Onions, chives and leeks also have similar, but lesser, benefits.

iii) Noni juice

Sadly the heavy marketing of this product, often bordering on the over claim, gets in the way of the real and excellent benefits of this natural fruit. I am a firm personal convert. It can be eaten as a fruit but is far more readily available as a concentrated fruit drink.

Firstly, it helps combat acid ash in the body, helping it achieve an alkaline pH, which is beneficial to all cellular biochemistry, and particularly the immune system in the fight against cancer.

Secondly, it has been shown in extensive research to promote a stronger immune system increasing the production of both B- and T-lymphocytes and to be a 'protector' against cancer. This is largely due to its content of polysaccharides (see glycoproteins Q21), which promote the immune system and aid its ability to identify rogue cells.

Noni contains a number of very potent alkaloids. For example, bromelain is known to weaken the walls of cancer cells and xeronine seems to help repair cells and in tests it produces a strong immune response against cancer cells. Noni also contains immune boosting polysaccharides in good quantities plus a variety of phytochemicals and Dr D L Davis, the senior science advisor to the US Public Health Service is very clear that, 'phytochemicals can take tumours and diffuse them'.

The Thais take it to aid digestion and avoid bacteria in the stomach and it can also be used to heal wounds and minor skin problems.

iv) Pau d'Arco

Pau d'Arco comes from the bark of a South American tree and has some anti-cancer activity due to the ingredient lapachol. It is a very powerful agent and originally was thought to have many direct effects on cancer. Due to the 20 or more active ingredients making it effective as an anti-fungal, antiviral, antibacterial and antimicrobial agent, it is now thought to be a very powerful, all-round body cleanser. This takes the pressure off the immune system so that the body can better restore full immune system power to fight the cancer.

It is widely used as a natural agent against parasites and candida and thus frees up the immune system to act fully in other areas.

v) Black cumin (*Nigella sativa*)

This is sometimes called cinnamon flower or nutmeg flower and is used for a variety of illnesses particularly in the Middle East.

Studies in 1991 by Nair showed extracts from the seeds to be toxic to cancer cells.

White blood cells treated with nigella seeds produce higher levels of interleukin plus a specific factor that stops the growth of tumours. Indeed two studies in 1997 and 1998, one by Medenica in the South Carolina, Immuno-Biology Research Laboratory and the other by Worthen both showed that the seeds inhibited tumour growth and the blood supply growth necessary for a tumour to form.

(vi) Essiac (sometimes called Cassie tea)

Sadly, this product, or rather blend of ingredients, is surrounded in mythology that tends to overshadow its real powers.

It was probably used by native American Indians for several hundred years as a herbal remedy in all sorts of illnesses. In 1922 a patient of Nurse Rene Caisse in Canada told her about a herbal infusion that had cured her breast cancer some 20 years before. Caisse saw the results for herself and incorporated the use of the remedy into her patients' treatments.

Over the following 50 or more years Rene Caisse ran a very successful free cancer clinic in Canada, then another in conjunction with several doctors, notably Dr Charles Brusch in New England. Although she had clinical X-rays and pathological proof of her results, the Canadian Government never officially approved the treatment. Her own view was that, 'if it doesn't actually cure cancer, it does afford significant relief.'

She treated her own 72 year old mother with the tea under the supervision of Dr Roscoe Graham, consultant and specialist. The tea was administered 12 times a day for 10 days, and her mother lived to 90 years of age.

The active ingredients were:

- **Burdock root** – a well known blood purifier which can decrease cell mutation and inhibit tumours. It has a reasonably high selenium content
- **Sheep sorrel** – a traditional and powerful Indian remedy for everything from eczema to ringworm; it does have an effect in herpes, ulcers and cancer seemingly by stimulating the

endocrine system. It needs to be prepared slowly and correctly to be effective.

- **Slippery elm** – calcium, magnesium and vitamin rich, it has a healing effect on the lungs and internal organs. It also helps reduce acid ash in the body.
- **Indian rhubarb** – very cleansing to the liver and intestinal system. It also helps transport oxygen throughout the body and has an antibiotic and anti-yeast action and reduces inflammation. In 1980 studies showed that it also had a clear anti-tumour effect.

Whilst working with Dr Brusch between 1959 and 1978, Nurse Caisse added four other herbs to the formula (the current formula is her name spelled backwards). The four additions are:

- **Watercress** – a powerful antioxidant, containing bioflavonoids; it is a good blood purifier.
- **Blessed thistle** – a blood purifier and immune booster
- **Red clover** – the herb of Hippocrates, the flowers are currently undergoing tests in the UK for breast cancer control.
- **Kelp** – like chlorophyll and spirolina, kelp is a strong provider of natural minerals especially iron and calcium in an organic and easily assimilated form. Kelp is antibacterial and sea vegetables, in general, help reduce acidity in the body thus improving immune function.

Nurse Caisse recommended 12–13 cups of the infusion per day. Shortly before she died she sold the 'secret' formula to a company called Resperin.

(vii) Hoxsey's formula

Hoxsey was dubbed 'The quack who cured cancer' by a reporter who spent six weeks in 1939 reviewing Hoxsey's work in Texas. It had all started with Hoxsey's father, a sick horse and an observation about herbs that the horse chose to eat in the field, herbs that subsequently cured the animal. Hoxsey developed his herbal formula and treated some 12,000 people before being shut down in the 1950's. The FDA took the view that he was a quack and that none of the herbs had any anti-cancer properties. However they did no tests on any part of the therapy. The Fitzgerald report to Congress and a 1988 OTA report both concluded that there was merit in Hoxsey's work and that there had been a positive conspiracy against him.

His herbs included:

Cascar
Poke Root
Burdock Root
Berberis Root
Buckthorn Bark
Stilingia Root
Prickly Ash Bark.

Other additives like potassium iodide or red clover were also used from time to time.

Recent research literature now confirms that all the herbs have potency. (Pokeweed stimulates the immune system to increase lymphocytes and immunoglobulin; burdock has 'considerable' anti-tumour activity as has burbery and buckthorn. Even the least studied herbs like prickly ash have anti-inflammatory benefits). Dr James Burke of the US Dept of Agriculture has confirmed this.

Hoxsey's work continues in a day clinic, the Bio-Medical Centre, in Mexico. External cancers are most frequently treated as are cancers of the blood. Ironically Hoxsey himself died of prostate cancer. And, yes, he did treat himself with his own formula, which just shows that with cancer treatments there are no guarantees!

(viii) Echinacea

Originally in the 16th and 17th centuries, echinacea was used by native Americans for just about every medical need. This flower has a number of active ingredients but its usage was surpassed by antibiotics, although it is now having a renaissance as an immune booster against colds and flu.

Echinacea (or purple coneflower) is a native plant to America and was first used officially in medical practices in 1887. Most researched in Germany, it boosts the immune system directly and particularly aids the ingestion of foreign particles by the white cells. It also directly attacks viruses. Whilst it is most used for helping in infections of the upper respiratory tract (e.g. colds, where it helps both prevent and shorten the duration), it does have several anti-cancer benefits.

It can reduce secondary infection after radiotherapy and chemotherapy. There is also some evidence that it helps reduce the rate of growth of brain tumours and it appears (according to the University of Munich) to stimulate interleukin and the production of white cells, increasing both T- and B-lymphocytes, the former by 30 per cent. Another study showed that it has a direct effect on interferon production, which in turn disrupts the genetic code of foreign particles like viruses and probably even cancer cells.

Whilst it does strengthen the immune system it should not be taken in the long term as it thins the blood. Six to eight weeks is the recommended maximum period.

In a paper by M J Verhoef (1999) *Neurology* vol. 52, echinacea was studied as an alternative therapy for neurological disease and in brain tumour patients with some successful results. 1,200 mgs is a normal daily dose.

(ix) Green tea

You should drink green tea every day. It contains many anti-oxidant polyphenols, especially catechins, which have been shown to inhibit the spread of cancer (*Nature* 1997; Jankun). According to Perth University (**icon** – November 2003) drinking green tea reduces prostate cancer risk by 33 per cent. In 2002 the same group showed drinking just one cup per day reduced ovarian cancer risk by 60 per cent.

In 2004 the prestigious Mayo Clinic completed their own research study on green tea and concluded that '4–7 cups per day stopped leukaemia in its tracks'.

Green tea seems to have a positive effect with people on radio-therapy and chemotherapy. It has also emerged as a leading candidate for the prevention of UV-induced skin cancer. And, if that's not enough, apparently green tea also helps you slim and evens out skin tone and wrinkles!

(x) Ginseng

Ginseng has energy inducing properties, some of which come from its caffeine content. However, it also has anti-cancer properties.

There are principally two types of ginseng:

- *Panax:* Oriental, Asiatic, Chinese, Korean or Japanese; although, increasingly, the Americans claim to grow the most effective varieties. The active ingredients in the roots are the phytochemical group Ginsenosides, specifically Rg1 and Rb1.
- *Siberian:* This is a completely different plant from the rain-forests of Northern China. The active phytochemicals are called Eleutheroides.

Panax appears to be the more relevant in cancer treatment. The active ingredients stimulate the production of interleukin and boost B- and T-lymphocytes and macrophages. There is some evidence that it boosts spleen cells to become active killers of cancer cells. In mice with lung cancer it reduces tumours by 44 per cent.

It also plays a part in relieving and preventing prostate cancer. Ginseng (Panax) should not be taken during radiotherapy or chemotherapy because it can result in decreased blood platelet clotting and bleeding.

(xi) Cat's claw (Uno de Gato)

Alkaloids are powerful substances found in certain herbs and plants. There are six such oxindole alkaloids in Uno de Gato bark.

This natural substance is found mainly in the Peruvian Rain Forest and China. It is known to be antiviral, anti-inflammatory, an antioxidant and an immune stimulator. Four of the alkaloids in particular help in phagocytosis, attacking, wrapping up and removing harmful organisms, viruses, antigens and rogue cells.

The herb has been shown to be very powerful in its use with both cancer and AIDS, and it is very beneficial in relieving side effects from both radio and chemotherapy.

You should take 1 gm per day on an empty stomach. It can also be drunk as a tea using 300 mgs per cup.

As an anti-cancer aid it is combined with wild yam and aloe vera, the combination being a very strong antiviral, anti-bacterial force and having a very strong synergistic effect on the immune system.

Cat's claw is a good supplement if you want to return your white cells to their top level after the debilitating effects of chemo or radiotherapy.

(xii) Salicylic acid

You may know this best as aspirin. But you don't have to take pills to derive the same benefits, you can eat almonds or take aloe vera, for example. In the 19th century people used to chew willow bark because of its anti-inflammatory benefits.

Inflammation has been shown to be a precursor in a number of cancers. The Mayo Clinic in 2000 showed that 81 mgs of aspirin per day (about a sixth of one tablet) could cut cancer rates (e.g. prostate, colon) by 40 to 50 per cent. Its anti-inflammatory activities also reduce the size of intestinal, pre-cancerous polyps. Recent research reported by the American Medical Association suggested it could cut breast cancer risk by 29 per cent and even lower oestrogen levels! Of course to those who have read the chapter on eicosanoids and John Vane, this is hardly new news.

Aspirin can cause stomach problems and there are even reports on dependency, so instead you may like to use ...

(xiii) Aloe vera

Used by people like the Egyptians and Ancient Greeks for burns, wounds, bites and skin problems, it is only in recent years its full benefits are starting to become clearer. The two principle actions of the 'ingredients' are immune system boosting – it improves levels of T-cells and interferon, and has been shown to stimulate tumour necrosis factor, shutting off the blood supply to tumours – and ingredients like salicylate, gamma-linoleic, gibberlin, sterols and the amino acids phenylalanine and tryptophan all have anti-inflammatory benefits.

It is also anti-viral and anti-bacterial in its action.

The immune system effects are largely due to its polysaccharide content (see 'glycoproteins') and one in particular, acetyl mannose, has been shown to provoke a strong immune response through cytokine action.

(xiv) Neem

Neem is a tree native to Burma, but widely found throughout India. Many parts of the tree are used in treatments – leaves, bark, roots – all with slightly different properties but so much so that neem is ofter called 'the village pharmacy'. The National Research Council in Washington DC said it was one fo the most promising of all plants and might actually benefit every person on the planet.

Rather like Pau d'Arco, there were claims for it originally as a 'cancer cure'. In fact it is strongly anti-fungal, anti-bacterial and anti-viral. It also seems to reduce blood sugar levels and helps with eradication of yeasts.

(xv) Carctol

This is a blend of eight Indian herbs formulated by Dr Nandlal Tiwari in India. He uses it as a cancer treatment and there are 'clinical studies' (albeit at levels that would not necessarily please all the powers that be in the Western health services) showing that people on orthodox treatments such as chemotherapy have much greater survival times and success in beating cancers.

Carctol is recommended to be taken in conjunction with a strict vegetarian, low salt, low sugar diet which is very alkalising. This type of diet can anyway be very helpful to cancer patients (see *The Tree of Life: The Anti-Cancer Diet*), so it is very hard to separate out the claims of the carctol alone. The formula certainly has its followers and the test results are impressive.

Carctol needs to be prescribed by a doctor.

(xvi) Wormwood

Wormwood Artemisia has two effects in relation to cancer.

First, it is strongly anti-parasitical and anti-fungal. It is favoured by a number of alternative practitioners as the best eradicator of parasites. In some cases it need only be taken for a few days, such is its effect, although there are concerns that it is mildly addictive.

Second, recent research suggests that within cells it is mildly oxidative and since oxygen is the enemy is the enemy of a cancer cell, it can cause the destruction of cancer itself.

(xvii) Indole 3 Carbinol

A compound that naturally occurs in broccoli, brussel sprouts, cabbage and other cruciferous vegetables it is known to reduce the risk of prostate, colon and breast cancers. Research convered in **icon** also shows that it is has been used in cases of prostate cancer for treatment, as it boosts certain enzymes that reduce malignancy.

In breast cancer research I3C was shown to convert oestrogen into its weaker sister oestrone, and this was confirmed in studies on prostate cancer.

Other research (*Journal of Biochemistry* February 1998) suggests I3C turns off an enzyme, which normally drives cell division.

Apart from eating lots of broccoli, there are supplements that can be taken.

(xviii) Mistletoe

There is a lot of scientific research coming from Germany on this naturally occurring parasite. In fact work started just after the First World War!

Its primary action is to boost the immune system and particularly the lymphroytes. However there is significant research evidence that it both kills cancer cells and stifles the blood system required for tumour growth.

It is claimed to be potent with both primary and secondary brain tumours. Various 'brands' have been formulated, Iscador being available in the UK. It needs to be prescribed by a doctor and initially is likely to cause flu-like symptoms, which may be severe. For more information see www.iconmag.co.uk

---

Please note: There is no doubt that these herbs are powerful additions to your anti-cancer armoury. Your doctor needs to know exactly what you are taking lest it interferes with recommended drugs. However, if he tells you to stop taking a herb, it is absolutely imperative you ask for the evidence and references for the study. Too much mythology and subjective opinion abounds.

Q21. Are there any other dietary factors that might help prevent or control a cancer?

All of the following help in the fight against cancer:

(i) Soy or soya

In July 2002 Cancer Research UK published findings on the clear benefits of soya. A study involving two pieces of research, the US National Cancer Institute and the University of Singapore concluded that women who consumed the most soya were 60 per cent less likely to have risky, dense breast tissue than those consuming little soya.

Soya contains substances that are positive cancer protectors. Chemicals called phytoestrogens in soya actually block the effect of animal oestrogen in breast and prostate cancers by blocking receptors on the cell surface where oestrogen can alight and promote cancer growth. The anti-breast cancer drug Tamoxifen acts in the same way, but has notable side effects. The receptors on the cell surface will accept any oestrogen, animal or plant.

One soya phytoestrogen, genistein, has been specifically shown to block mammary tumours in animals, and also to prevent the growth of the blood supply to all tumours. (This blood supply is essential for a tumour's growth.) Asian women can have up to 1,000 times more genistein in their blood than Western women. Professor Trevor Powles of the Royal Marsden describes genistein as an 'anti-oestrogen'. There is evidence that soya can repair sun damage and lighten pigmentation spots.

Soya should ideally be organically grown and non-GM. Avoid soya products like mass-produced soy sauce because of the additives it contains and look for miso soup, tofu and tempeh. Soya milk and yoghurts can be bought in health food shops and consumed instead of milk and milk yoghurts. Soya protein can be used instead of meat and miso soup is high in the anti-cancer health food list. Soya beans themselves are a terrific source of vitamin E.

It is estimated that the equivalent of two and a half bowls of soya milk per day provides a start level for strengthening and protection, but 30–100 gms per day is the ideal amount. You can supplement further with soya isoflavones in capsules.

The question everybody has to ask themselves is, 'why use milk, which has severe question marks hanging over it, when soya is actually a cancer protector?' The majority of people in the world do not use dairy products, or use them sparingly, so on a volume basis, milk is actually a substitute for soya in the world, not the other way round!

Soya does have its critics but some criticisms are factually inaccurate.

It is claimed that soya contains 10 times the aluminium of milk; this is not true, they are roughly the same. It is linked to allergies, particularly child allergies. This is probably because it was only introduced into the Western diet in the 1960's. It is claimed that consumption is actually very limited in the Far East. Anyone who has travelled there will know that beans are regularly consumed and a regular Chinese breakfast is rice in soya milk. Finally, people site the Gerson Institute who do not recommend it. I spoke with Charlotte Gerson about this. Dr Max Gerson avoided the use of soya simply because he wanted his patients to eat no protein or fat. Now Charlotte Gerson frowns on it, as it contains phytic acid which can inhibit the uptake of some minerals, the very cornerstone of the Gerson Therapy (Q25). They also avoid all pulses and green beans for this reason. Interestingly, the Plaskett therapy which updates and modernises Gerson from a scientific nutritional and biochemical basis, does use some soya with oestrogen driven cancers.

Soya is an incomplete protein containing, for example, no B-12 which needs to be provided by other sources after week eight.

Another generalism is that it is a non-argument to suggest that high soya consumption in the Far East is linked to low cancer rates because so many other local factors aid the population's health. Curiously many of the same people argue that the consumption of B-17 by Hunzas is uniquely linked to their low cancer rates!

Clearly the truth is that soya consumption is just a part of a diet that contains many vegetables and rice. The sensible solution is to understand that you cannot simply bring one element of a Far East diet to the West and expect it to 'work'. But it might just help!

(ii) Other isoflavones

Beans, lentils, chickpeas, many vegetables and legumes all contain good levels of isoflavones as do herbs such as red clover blossoms, which were used by many ancient herbalists. Tests are currently taking place at The Royal Marsden Hospital to see if red clover can actually prevent breast cancer.

These foods are not just important for their phytoestrogen but the fact that their fibre content in the gut actually aids the disposal of, for example, excess oestrogen hormone from the body. In 1900 up to 30 per cent of protein in the British diet came from pulses (beans, peas, lentils). Now it is less than 2 per cent. We are no longer eating foods that best protect us.

(iii) Fish oils

Fish oils contain vitamin A, vitamin D and high levels of long chain omega 3 fatty acids, as covered in the piece on eicosanoids. They are the ultimate 'triple whammy' in the fight against cancer. However, all fish oils were not created equal. Cod liver oil has the highest levels of omega 3 but little vitamin D. Either mix cod liver oil and general fish oils, or look for a cod liver oil supplemented with vitamin D. Although oils generally tend to encourage cancer development, omega 3 seems to stop the spread of cancer cells, probably by binding to cell membranes to protect healthy cells and inhibit cancer cells. Tests on mice with fish oils showed a reduction in spread of cancer tumours by 60 per cent. In one test omega 3 stopped the production of prostaglandins – hormone like substances that encourage cancer and poor cell division. Omega 3 oils replace and balance out omega 6 and other oils (notably saturated fats and cooking oils, somewhat typically, used in fast foods).

Walnut oil, olive oil, flaxseed oil and macadamia nut oil all contain omega 3 fatty acids but these are the short chain version and seem to be neutral in the body. Only about 14 per cent of short-chain converts to long-chain. As explained before, you should avoid taking too much cod liver oil as a supplement because of the possible overload on the body of vitamin A. 1,000 mgs once per day is the upper limit and even then you should have rest periods.

However, if you had to take three supplements to beat cancer and generally improve your health, they should be fish oils, fish oils and fish oils.

Dioxins and toxins are a problem in certain fish oils. Look for 'pure' fish oils where possible.

(iv) Glutathione

Glutathione is a very powerful antioxidant that helps neutralise rancid fats. It is a naturally occurring amino acid but the body can make it as well. Studies show clearly that, in older people those with the highest blood levels overcome illness quickest.

Glutathione is produced in all cells of the body, specifically to break down dangerous toxins and free radicals. It works in the gut, in the blood stream and in the cells. Its particular strength is with peroxides, the precursors of free radicals, and also with bad fats.

Brussel sprouts, cabbage, cauliflower and broccoli are the usual recommended providers but top of the list are avocado, asparagus, watermelon, grapefruit, boiled potatoes, strawberries, raw tomatoes, oranges, and orange juice.

You can take 100 mgs of glutathione with your meal. Also taking glutamine, an amino acid supplement, pumps up glutathione in the body and boosts the immune system. It can be taken as two teaspoons of glutamine powder (8,000 mgs) daily dissolved in water. Two to three times that volume may be needed if you are ill.

German work stemming from a 1998 Nobel Prize has shown that toxic cells lose their energy-producing ability and 'power down'. Below certain levels of power, protective genes cannot work. Glutathione levels seem to be very important in keeping cellular energy high. Some alternative cancer therapists focus on low glutathione levels found in the cells of cancer patients, trying to drive them, and thus oxygen levels, upwards.

(v) Cysteine and cystine

Cystine is the stable form of a sulphur-based amino acid called cysteine. The body converts between the two. By taking the supplement L-cystine with vitamin C in a 1:3 ratio with food you can add further protection against free radical damage – particularly that from smoking, drinking and X-ray radiation. It also works to detoxify, and counter balance the carcinogenic factor homo-cysteine.

(vi) Shark cartilage

'Sharks don't get cancer', so the story goes. Sharks have no bones, only flexible cartilage. By taking this cartilage and pummelling it carefully, so that it breaks down without disrupting the active protein chains, treatments have been prepared from the resulting powder. As with soya isoflavones and garlic, the action of the protein is claimed to prevent or reduce the growth of cancers. It does this by restricting the blood supply to the cancer, called angeniosis (remember a tumour over 1cm needs its own blood supply). However after positive TV documentaries in the USA, many firms rushed out capsules. Critics claim that, even if these contained the right purified active ingredient, cancer sufferers would need to take almost a whole bottle per day.

It is however used by some clinics in its correct and pure form and apparently does have a positive effect.

(vii) Acidophilus

Lactobacillus acidophilus is a source of friendly intestinal bacteria. The friendly bacteria in the gut weigh in total about 1.5 kilos, and they are the first line of defence in the immune system. Antibiotics, steroids, statins, chemotherapy and even chlorine from tap water seem to destroy friendly natives in the intestine, allowing an overgrowth of fungus microbes and yeasts to occur.

Lactose, pectin and vitamin C aid the growth of 'friendlies' (lactose is, however, a milk sugar). Acidophilus unfortunately can die off in just three days if your body is unbalanced or stressed, so topping up the bacteria on a regular basis is an insurance policy, especially since if the yeast fungus takes over it leaches vitamins, particularly B vitamins, and minerals from the system. Acidophilus is also known to keep Helicobacter pylori in check.

There is some indication that acidophilus, in standard pill form, may be destroyed by the pH in the stomach, thus preventing it from reaching the intestines. Slow release pills are apparently the answer to this problem.

If it is possible that you are susceptible to this type of yeast infection, you should avoid eating live bakers yeast and B complex vitamins with yeast.

There is some evidence that small pieces of the cell walls of friendly bacteria can pass through the lining of the intestine into the blood system. In tests, these bacteria wall pieces kill cancer cells.

(viii) Red wine

Red grapes, particularly cabernet grapes, contain high concentrations of catechins in their skins. Catechins block tumours and oxidative free radicals and inhibit bacteria and viruses. Red wine has glycoprotein activity – see later – and a strong natural antioxidant called resveratrol. One glass of cabernet sauvignon twice a week would be helpful. No more mind! You can have too much of a good thing.

(ix) Eating less calories than you need

You may have read about the rats that were fed 40 per cent less food and lived to the equivalent of 140 years of age. There are huge benefits in calorie restriction for humans too:

- Eating too much bombards your cells with free radicals. The less calories you consume, the less energy is made in the power stations in your cells, so the less waste toxins and free radicals you produce. An excess of free radicals affects the balance of your various hormones and reduces communication between them.
- Calorie restriction causes an increase in protective enzymes and, if it occurs over a lengthy and continuous period, stimulates the production of melatonin and human growth hormone both of which neutralise free radicals.
- Calorie restriction reduces the likelihood of excess insulin production and less insulin means less bad eicosanoids. It also

reduces excess blood glucose, known to damage the hypothalamus, the control centre for all hormones.

So it's not just the rats that benefit. In the war the Germans took away much of the Norwegians' food, leaving them on a calorie restricted diet with a high fish content. During those five years the heart attack rate fell significantly.

There is further evidence that eating less reduces the cancer risk in humans. The Okinawans have a calorie-restricted diet. They eat three times more vegetables and twice as much fish as the average Japanese but far less rice, animal protein, and fat resulting in a healthier diet but also a consumption of about 20–40 per cent less calories. They eat virtually no salt.

Their cancer rate is 60 per cent less. They have the highest longevity rates in the world.

(x) Polysaccharides and glycoproteins

Over the last seven years, four Nobel Prizes in physiology and medicine have gone to people looking at, for example, how the brain communicates with cells or how cells themselves communicate. When the nuclear DNA wants to direct your body to make green eyes or five toes it makes a protein message. But it has to tag this message with a post-code so that it ends up in the right destination.

In 1999 Dr Gunter Blobel won the Nobel Prize for showing how the protein messages have this post-code in them, how they pass across protein cell walls, and how errors in this system can be linked to cancer, AIDS, the herpes virus and hereditary diseases. In 2001, Hartwell, Hunt and Nurse won a Nobel Prize for showing an understanding on the cellular messages involved in the cell cycle – its growth and division into two identical daughter cells – and how mistakes might result in a cancer development..

Some of this work had led already to drugs being produced, and one alone Arithroprotein, is a $2 bn business in the USA.

Certain polysaccharides and glycoproteins (special protein/ sugar like compounds) seem to have a role in helping this message system work effectively. They can improve the quality of the messages; they can 'clean up' your cell membranes and particularly receptor sites so that viruses and bacteria have more problems launching their attacks; and they can help your T-cells 'spot' a rogue cell amongst the healthy ones. They also boost many aspects of the immune system.

Sources for these saccharides include Japanese and Chinese mushrooms, onions, garlic, shellfish, bovine cartilage, breast milk, pectins (apples and citrus fruit eaten whole), noni juice, aloe vera and arabinogalactins (in corn, leeks, radishes, peas, red wine, coconut, curcumin, rice, psyllium, echinacea, tomatoes, carrots and the bark of certain trees). Aloe vera polysaccharides have been shown to stop bacteria and viruses actually binding to and infecting cells.

Shitake, maitake, reishi and cordycep mushrooms have been shown to have anti-cancer properties. Medicinal mushrooms contain bio-available beta glucan polysaccharide which is a proven anti-mutagen (ie stops the formation of the first rogue); it increases apoptosis and reduces skin cancer in mice. The use of mushroom nutrition is standard practice in many orthodox Japanese cancer treatments.

In a recent paper from Strathclyde University medicinal mushrooms also improved immune system strength, reduced side effects of both radio and chemotherapy, improved the quality of life amongst long-term cancer patients and improved survival rates.

A survey in one region of Japan, and covered in November 2002 by Cancer Research UK, showed that the mushroom pickers had 66 per cent less cancer than the surrounding population. 'Scrumping' has its benefits!

Certain important developments have already come from this work. Coriolus mushrooms, which have been shown to activate T-lymphocytes, macrophages and other white cell immune factors is used as a treatment for cancer. Reishi has been widely studied and is available as a supplement. Maitake supplements have been shown in the Kobe College of Pharmacy, Japan, to increase the body's ability to destroy tumours.

And probably the most interesting supplement is MGN-3 (which is now branded Biobran in the UK). This has quite extensive research to support its immune system boosting claims including clinical trials. It appears to reduce side effects during chemotherapy and radiotherapy, and boost success rates for both. It is taken as a supplement but is quite expensive on a daily basis. Its activity seems to kick-in after about one month.

Another strong polysaccharide mix, used by a number of alternative cancer specialists is the brand Ambrotose, from Mannetech.

Only recently a professor of oncology told me that glyco-proteins and polysaccharides would be bigger than all the discoveries on vitamin C, B-17 and genistein added together! Together with other natural compounds and vitamins they can improve the quantity of the immune system. But their special powers seem to lie in improving the quality of the immune system too.

In a cancer patient only one in a thousand T-cells might 'work' – glycoproteins can get those T-cells working again and spotting the rogue cells. Exactly what every cancer patient needs!

Q22. Learn to eat properly!

Ask any woman who has bad pre-menstrual pains how rapidly they are eased by evening primrose oil; or over-eat beetroot or asparagus and see how quickly your urine is affected. What you eat and drink affects your body quite rapidly, so it is wise to eat properly. Here are a few tips:

- If vegetables are eaten raw at the start of a meal (e.g. crudités, or raw vegetables with some dips), up to 40 per cent more vitamins and minerals are absorbed.
- Consumption of water before, during or at the end of the meal should be avoided. Excess water merely dilutes the digestive enzymes and prevents them from working fully. Drink copious amounts of water but at least one and a half hours from a meal.
- Eat slowly and focus on the food. Reading, working or watching TV can cause a whole range of emotions and stress to alter your hormone balance and prevent the perfect uptake of vitamins and minerals.
- Chew thoroughly. This releases an enzyme in the saliva called ptyalin which is crucial to the proper digestion of carbohydrates. Try and eat four to six small meals per day to maintain your blood sugar levels and put less strain on your digestive tract and endocrine system.
- Do not eat carbohydrate and protein at the same time. In the wild, our natural environment saw us find tubers and eat them, or gorge at a fruit tree, or capture an animal. We didn't take them all back to the cave and eat them on the same plate! Your digestive system is not designed for this total simultaneous consumption.

  The carbohydrate and ptyalin mixture passes to the stomach where it needs an alkaline environment for maximum efficiency. Carbohydrate on its own clears the stomach in about one hour.

  Protein on the other hand passes to the stomach where it meets its digestive enzyme pepsin and this requires an acid environment. Protein on its own can be digested in about one and a half hours.

But mix the two and the stomach doesn't know whether to be alkaline or acid, with the result that the food is improperly digested and takes up to eight hours to pass through. This results in inefficiency throughout the intestinal system.

Worse, after the age of 50, humans steadily produce less and less acid making food separation even more critical for proper nourishment and digestion.

- In our Western world, where most of us have yeast infections, fruits should always be consumed first, at the start of the meal and on an empty stomach. Otherwise they can sit on top of a meal and ferment, causing toxins to be produced. People on anti-yeast diets need to avoid this complication as the fermentation aids the growth of yeasts.

- Vegetables, pulses, and oats, for example, contain soluble fibre. This is essential to the alimentary canal where it dissolves, transports, and helps excrete toxins and excess hormones. Rice should be eaten at least once a day (preferably organic whole and brown), as it is particularly good at cleaning your system.

- Eat fresh vegetables, fresh herbs, and fresh fruit. And try to eat them as close to the raw state as possible. Raw or steamed vegetables retain their nourishment values best, whilst boiling tends to reduce vitamin and mineral levels. But you don't just get vitamins and minerals from vegetables. When you pick broccoli it has an energy field, an aura. Despite steaming, broccoli retains most of this energy and the aura can still be seen in special photographs. If you microwave broccoli almost all the energy and aura is lost. Little work has been done on this subject but quite possibly our absorption of the energy of our foodstuffs is as important as the vitamin and mineral content.

- Restrict meat and fish to four times per week. Have vegetarian days. Pulses are an excellent protein source for these non-meat days. Why have non-meat days? I have already talked about animal fats. In a research study on women in northern Italy commissioned by New York University, two similar groups of women were studied, both of which ate lots of carbohydrate and olive oil, but the group consuming meat and dairy had three times the cancer risk.

- If a woman cuts her fat intake in half, her oestrogen level will fall 20 per cent or more.
- Because fat is a good solvent, animal fat actually accumulates toxins the animal ate or produced. Meat and fish also bring their hormones into your body.
- Cooking meat produces carcinogens. The most dangerous is the production of nitrosamines from meat being burnt, or from the smoke of the coals or wood, on barbecues. Even when animal proteins are heated they produce heterocyclic amines and grilled chicken is 15 times worse than beef! (Sinha, Rothman, Brown (1995) *Cancer Research*).
- The World Health Organisation (WHO) has recently confirmed that acrylamides cause cancer. In January 2002, acrylamides were found by Swedish researchers in chips, crisps, breakfast cereals, crispbreads, biscuits, and other foods cooked (usually baked) at very high temperatures.
- Fried food in general is bad for you. Fried meat is linked to a higher risk of hormone related cancers in women, and men who eat fried food regularly have a three times higher risk than people who eat it in moderation.
- Stomach cancer is linked with smoked, pickled, salted or dried foods, where sodium nitrite is used as a preserving agent.
- Cut salt. As we keep saying. Never add salt, and avoid all foods that may contain it as a preservative or taste enhancer. (Chinese meals with MSG can give you 10–15gms in one sitting!!)
- Pickled foods, alcohol and tobacco increase cancer risk in the oesophagus. Meat, alcohol and coffee are turning the previously low rates of pancreatic cancer in Japan into Western numbers.
- In 2004 The Soil Association reviewed 21 foods and showed that in organic foods on average, vitamin C levels were 27 per cent higher and magnesium 29 per cent higher, for example.
- A review of pesticide residues in the USA showed that

certain foods (sadly the red and yellow ones like peppers, strawberries and cherries) are more likely to accumulate pesticides. A full review is available on www.iconmag.co.uk.

I hope you find this list of 'tips' helpful. Eating properly requires effort and time. Don't bring certain foods into the house in the first place; modify your cooking and eating habits and start all your planning with fruit and vegetables.

Remember the well-worn cliché: You are what you eat. Never is it more true than in cancer.

Q23. Which natural foods offer the best sources of the important vitamins and minerals?

If the UK Government's recommendation is that you should eat five helpings of fresh fruit and vegetables a day, what is a helping? If someone has five boiled potatoes, is that the Government's view of providing daily health? The US Government in their wisdom decreed in June 2004 that a portion of French Fries actually counts as a vegetable!! But is that really sensible?

Meanwhile, the French Government wants its population to eat 10 portions. And the recent US health directive for the American population has suggested 13 portions of fruit and vegetables per day is the aim. Who is right and where is the justification for this?

First, governments have to be well researched, well argued and clear on their recommendations and make them less woolly and more relevant to the population. Then a total education programme needs to be started, in schools and through advertising and PR, which encourages children and their parents to understand what is really being recommended and why.

But in the short term, where do you go to provide a good diet with the required levels of, say, antioxidants? Well, often it is not the fruit and veg. Here is a simple guide to some of the best natural sources of each vitamin or mineral in the fight against cancer:

Vitamin E

2 tablespoons of sunflower seeds	11 mgs
1 tablespoon sunflower oil	6 mgs
20 almonds	8 mgs
1 tablespoon of soya oil	3 mgs
1 tablespoon of wheatgerm	3 mgs

You can see from this that it is hard to get near the ideal level of 400 IU of vitamin E naturally per day (400 IU = 268 mgs) without taking vitamin supplements. Throw sunflower seeds on salads, have a bowl of pumpkin, sunflower and sesame seeds to nibble rather than crisps or peanuts.

Vitamin C

1 large red pepper	224 mgs
100 gms raw broccoli	90 mgs
150 gms papaya	90 mgs
1 large orange	65 mgs

Surprisingly then the top vitamin C producer is not an orange! Your morning glass of orange juice only gives you about 10 mgs and is usually pasteurised and full of sugar unless you have squeezed it yourself. So it's chopped red pepper with everything and broccoli as raw as possible (but wash it well).

Beta-carotene

1 cup carrot juice	24.2 mgs
1 medium sweet potato	10.0 mgs
5 dried apricots	6.2 mgs
1 cup red cherries	6.2 mgs
½ cup cooked spinach	5.7 mgs
1 cup tomato juice	2.2 mgs

Beta-carotene is plentiful in nature in colourful foods and green vegetables. Red and yellow peppers, tomatoes and kale are others.

Lycopene

1 standard tin of tomato soup	65 mgs
1 tin of vegetable juice	23 mgs
5 tablespoons of tomato paste	22 mgs
5 tablespoons of tomato ketchup	12 mgs

So you need to look little further than tomatoes. The next best are watermelons. Studies show men who eat seven servings a week of tomatoes and tomato products reduce their prostate risk by 40 per cent. Cooked tomatoes are best as they release their lycopene more easily to your digestive system.

Zinc

6 oysters	55 mgs
Medium serving of steak	8 mgs
4 tablespoons of sunflower seeds	6 mgs
Serving of All Bran	4 mgs

Well it's oysters every day now! Zinc is ubiquitous and you are only trying to get to 15–25 mgs per day.

Selenium

4 cracked brazil nuts in shells	150 mcgs
4 slices of wholemeal bread	60 mcgs
2 tablespoons sunflower seeds	15 mcgs
1 egg	15 mcgs
1 skinless chicken breast	10 mcgs

Try to avoid brazil nuts (or any nuts) in cellophane wrappers as depending upon their shelf time they may be rancid. Crack them yourself.

Omega 3 fatty acids

Salmon	1.0 mgs per gm
Herring	1.0 mgs per gm
Mackerel	0.9 mgs per gm

As we covered with eicosanoids, fish oils provide omega 3 in a most concentrated form. Mackerel wins in terms of overall health because it has least total fat.

Calcium

100 gms tinned sardines	460 mgs
100 gms almonds	250 mgs

By comparison a glass of skimmed milk gives only 120 mgs and 150 gm low fat yoghurt gives 190 mgs.

Just from this brief study you can see how easy it is to reach your targets, and that is without the five helpings of fruit and vegetables a day, although they do play a crucial role with the fibre you need.

Q24. Are there any specific diets that could be useful?

Before we get into specific diets, there are a couple of possible additions to the anti-cancer armoury that are worth knowing.

(a) The juice fast

Dr Otto Buchinger Jr is considered by many to be the leading expert in this area and he calls juice fasts, 'the royal road to healing'. Using a good juicer and organically grown produce, you first soak the fruit and vegetables in a big bowl of water containing 1 capful of peroxide to remove bacteria, chemical residues and parasites.

Raw juices like carrot, beetroot, celery, cabbage, apple, and watercress can be surprisingly tasty. Add a little ginger to help the taste if you wish. They are extremely cleansing, easy to digest, and packed full of vitamins, minerals and enzymes.

The detoxification process, which should be used for three to seven days, may result at first in some side effects like headaches, bad breath, tiredness, dizziness and even memory loss but health comes back with a vengeance.

The fast can be helped by:

- Liver cleansers like milk-thistle and other herbs;
- Colon cleansers like psyllium, alfalfa, goldenseal, and slippery elm.
- Aloe vera which helps kill bacteria, viruses, yeasts and helps to heal the damage from radiation and chemotherapy.
- Bromelain and papain, both of which are digestive enzymes that hit foreign substances including cancer cells.

You may also use blood cleansers like kelp, chlorella (which in particular binds heavy metals), and Essiac, which also helps to clean the liver and gallbladder and expel toxins in the gut. The latter is an excellent all round agent. Question 15 provides details on more general detoxing.

Immune system boosters can be taken at the same time. For example, echinacea which also cleans the blood and lymph systems, cat's claw and astralagus. (See Question 20)

133

(b) The coffee enema

You must be joking! No seriously, it has a very big fan club amongst alternative health doctors and practitioners. Enemas, like colonic irrigation, remove the toxins from the colon. The presence of organic coffee with caffeine stimulates the liver to cleanse itself (conversely actually drinking coffee poisons the whole system with caffeine) and opens up the bile ducts into the intestine. Stomach massage and castor oil also help clear out the toxins and prevent them being re-absorbed. The main draw back is that, with some cancer treatments, four enemas are recommended per day, each in all taking about 60–90 minutes. Coffee enemas are used by many of the major cancer clinics.

Diets

The principle of, 'You are what you eat' stems from naturopathy and the belief that we are at one with our surroundings. The opposite of health is illness. There is only one state of health and all illness is one; it is just represented in a number of forms. If cancer is brought on by poor nourishment, then good nourishment is the way to beat it.

(i) The macrobiotic diet

In Greek 'macro' means great, and 'biotic' means concerning life. Macrobiotics, or the greater view of life, is based on the ancient Chinese understanding of yin and yang in the universe and is not confined to diet at all. The Chinese believe that everything in the universe can be divided into these two categories (think mother or father aspect), although it is fluid and one form can change into the other.

Between 1896 and 1907 Sagen Ishizuka, a Japanese army doctor developed a theory of nutrition. In it he combined both the Western medical thinking with ancient Oriental thinking. His basic tenet was that the food we eat not only sustains life but underpins our health and happiness.

During this period of time Japan was being heavily Westernised and he argued strongly against it, recommending re-adoption of the traditional Japanese diet, ie. whole, unrefined foods with little or no milk or animal food. He set up a clinic and treated hundreds of patients with a traditional diet based on brown rice and a variety of land and sea vegetables. Such was his success that he became known as the 'Anti-Doctor'.

His five principles were:

1. Foods are the foundation of health and happiness
2. Sodium and potassium are opposites in food, and control its yin and yang character.
3. Grain is properly the staple food of man
4. Food should be unrefined, whole, and natural
5. Food should be grown locally and in season

Macrobiotic diets also require that foods are eaten as near the natural state as possible and cooking is almost an art form.

The use of a macrobiotic diet requires that there is an understanding of the patient's yin and yang state and that foods are then provided to correct any imbalance. The detail of their use for say the cancer patient, is beyond the scope of this book. You should telephone your local centre, contact the Macrobiotic Association and/or go to the website for a better understanding of how a macrobiotic diet might fit your personal needs. A fundamental part of macrobiotics is that everyone of us is different and one man's grain is another man's poison. So you must check it out thoroughly before you act on any advice. But the evidence is clear. A basic Japanese diet is much, much better for your health than a Western diet.

(ii) The Bristol Cancer Centre diet

This has been prepared for cancer sufferers by the Bristol Cancer Help Centre. It is not a diet therapy in its own right but guidelines and recommendations for a diet in support of other cancer treatments.

The guidelines suggest:

- consuming a large variety of fresh vegetables and fruits, especially raw
- increasing the range of grains you eat, especially wholegrain, to include quinoa, brown rice, barley and millet
- including beans and lentils at least three times per week and avoiding added bran

135

- eating nuts and seeds (sesame, sunflower, poppy, pumpkin).
- only using cold pressed plant oils for cooking and dressings (e.g. olive oil, sunflower oil)
- using freshly made organic fruit and vegetable juices where possible
- drinking 2 litres of filtered or bottled water per day.

Avoiding:

- red meat (beef, lamb or pork)
- saturated fat (milk, cream, cheese, yoghurt) – substituting soya
- smoked and salt cured foods
- refined sugar (use honey if necessary)
- processed and refined foods, which have preservatives.
- salt and sugar
- caffeine in coffee, tea, chocolate, and fizzy drinks
- excess alcohol
- sweet fizzy drinks.

The Bristol Cancer Centre also has courses covering meditation, visualisation and diet. It embraces holistic doctors, healers, nutritional therapists and counsellors.

(iii) Metabolic typing

There is an argument that severely challenges the 'vegetarian is best' doctrine and diets like that of the Bristol Cancer Centre in treating **all** cancer patients. The macrobiotic diet certainly does not hold that one diet fits all. As we will see in Q48, William Kelley in his cancer treatments identified that 'one man's meat really was another man's poison'. He showed there were a number of different metabolic and biochemical 'types' of people in the world. Some responded well to a strictly vegetarian diet whilst others needed meat. A more simple version of this is used in Dr Peter J D'Adamo's book *Eat Right for Your Type* which concerns just our blood types and their relation to our personal food needs. However a more comprehensive assessment using nine factors can be obtained over the net using a system developed by Bill Wolcott who worked with Kelley (www.healthexcel.com).

(iv) John Boik

John Boik works with the prestigious MD Anderson Cancer Institute in Texas. In March 2001 he published *Natural Compounds in Cancer Therapy* a tome that includes 4000 detailed scientific references. He divided the cancer process into stages and showed that for each stage (e.g. cell formation, cell division, metastasis, etc) there were natural compounds that could counter the cancer, from astragalus to vitamin E. His book, although awesome, is well worth reading if you choose to try to beat a cancer by the scientific use of diet. Frankly the book should be read by every oncologist in Britain as it clearly lays out the scientific evidence that foods, vitamins, minerals and herbs have a proven role to play in cancer treatment. There is now no excuse for dietary ignorance.

(v) Other

Closer to home, **Dr Etienne Callebout** is a Belgian doctor working in Harley Street. He uses a number of scientific tests (including comprehensive blood testing) to build a regenerative programme including diet. The diet will be individually tailored to your specific biochemistry and is thus his version of metabolic typing. Callebout also believes in enhancing the mental state and attitude of mind.

If you decide to follow an essentially vegetarian diet to help 'beat' your cancer, please pay attention to your vitamin levels particularly B-12 and vitamin A as shortfalls are linked with a number of cancers.

But all in all, it is quite clear that attention to your diet should be a primary factor in cancer prevention or cancer treatment. If nothing else surely there is a simple logic to this: If the World Health Organisation believes that half of all cancers are caused by poor diet is it not simply logical that at least **some** of these could be corrected by a good diet?

If you want to read more about the specific foods that might help you and about the underpinning science of diet therapies (but in an easy-to-understand way) try *The Tree of Life: The Anti-Cancer Diet*, my book specific to this subject.

Q25. What about diet therapies?

As we have said, the WHO believes at least 50 per cent of all cancers are caused by diet. Certainly the people who ring our office at the outset of their cancer seem to be both nutritionally deficient and nutritionally toxic.

Logic dictates that if some cancers are 'caused' by poor diet, might not at least some of these be corrected by a good diet?

The **Gerson Therapy** is based around the hourly consumption of freshly prepared organic juices, which not only detox, but keep up high vitamin and particularly mineral levels in the body re-establishing a healthy metabolism. It was developed by Dr Max Gerson who had a number of successful clinics. Dr Albert Schweitzer called him, 'one of medicine's most eminent geniuses'. Gerson died in 1959 so there is no doubt he was ahead of his time in suggesting certain causes of cancer and in his belief that you had to attack the cause not the symptoms.

This treatment is a whole body treatment incorporating the principles of detoxification of the wastes and toxins that interfere with healing and normal metabolism, and an intensive nutritional programme to flood the body with healing nutrients. Thirteen fresh organic juices are consumed everyday and enemas, including the coffee enema, are used to detox. The juices are made from over 20 pounds of organically grown nuts and vegetables daily; one glass, 13 times. Some organic vegetables and fruits are consumed whole. The metabolism is also stimulated by the addition of thyroid, potassium and other supplements.

Dr Max Gerson wrote up the results of 50 successful cancer cures in his original book *A Cancer Therapy: Results of 50 Cases*. He lived from 1881 to 1959 and was truly ahead of his time. His diet eliminates all free radicals where possible, protein, fats and excess sodium, whilst flooding the body with potassium and magnesium along with many, many fresh vitamins, minerals and enzymes. The therapy has its critics. Gerson's view that a natural diet would restore the body's resistance and healing power lost through years of artificial nutrition meant he openly criticised a lot of modern foods and these are banned from the diet, for example, dairy, wheat, caffeine, animal fat, excess protein, and sodium.

In July 2004 HRH Prince Charles expressed a view that alternative therapies such as the Gerson Therapy should be properly researched so that we could all have objective evidence on their success rates. He was immediately attacked by 'medical experts' who said things like, "How could coffee possibly cure cancer?" These comments merely highlighted their own ignorance as neither Gerson nor other diet therapists have ever suggested coffee as anything other than an agent to cause dilation of the bile ducts and something that aided the release of toxins into the intestine. Other attacks, of course, were made on the abuse of his royal role to 'meddle' in medicine.

But HRH was quite right. The truth is we do need accurate evidence on Gerson, Metabolic Therapy, Hoxsey and the like. Good or bad. As you will see later, one 'diet therapy' used by Gonzalez in New York, is being properly evaluated in 'clinical trials'. And it is surpassing all the results from chemotherapy treatment. But I'm on no one's side – I just want objective facts, as I suspect does everyone reading this.

The Gerson Institute is in San Diego, but Californian law does not permit them to treat patients there. They now have a clinic in Mexico and a centre in Liverpool, England. Qualified support groups exist on a more local basis.

The Gerson therapy can even be adopted at home, although proper medical supervision is recommended.

Dr Lawrence Plaskett in the UK is a long time admirer of the pioneering work of Gerson in the 1940s and 1950s. Dr Plaskett currently holds the vice-chair of the Nutritional Therapy Council in the UK.

Plaskett had long offered nutritional treatment in his practice and decided to design a new therapy based on a common medical philosophy with Gerson, but incorporating many of the newer nutritional discoveries and biochemical advances. Using his nutritional expertise and incorporating a lengthy and detailed study of the research literature available covering anti-carcinogenic and anti-tumour nutrients, foods and nutriceuticals, Plaskett developed a completely separate therapy.

The therapy consists of a very specific diet, nutritional supplement programme, herbs, juices, coffee enemas and even some complex naturopathic remedies. It embodies variations that take into account the differing needs of patients with cancers of different types.

Dr Plaskett now has a college which trains practitioners in nutritional medicine and he no longer treats patients these days. Instead, he has passed his therapy on to the National Cancer Therapy Trust (NCTT) for practical application in the UK. There are over 70 fully qualified practitioners working with the Trust throughout the UK, and since 1997 those patients who have been able to take the therapy fully and consistently have shown remarkable results.

Q26. Can screening help beat cancer?

All the best advice is that the earlier you discover a cancer the greater your odds are of beating it. Screening can play an important part in this process. However it is nowhere near as accurate as the medical profession would have us believe. Basically screening can be simplified under three headings.

(i) Tried and trusted methods?

Palpation (looking for a lump with your fingers)

Women over 30 should examine their **breasts** at least every month. In the USA if you have ever had radiation treatment on the chest region, it is recommended that start self-screening much earlier. The self-test should be performed seven to ten days after the start of the menstrual period, since the texture and density of the breast tissue will change during the monthly cycle. Women who are post-menopausal should choose the same day every month.

Firstly conduct a visual examination studying the size, dimpling, and shape of each breast including the nipple. Then gently feel your breasts using the pads of your three longest fingers looking for lumps, bumps and changes. A fuller description can be obtained from the breast cancer charity (see Appendix for contact details).

Mammography

Years of usage of the mammogram, especially in the USA, has created a popular belief in its importance. And during the 70s and 80s as mammograms came into widespread use, coupled with early detection and a greater consciousness of breast cancer, breast cancer deaths fell by 30 per cent.

Mammograms provide a detailed image of the breast tissue. If the tissue is soft, detection of an unusual lump is relatively easy, but becomes harder the more 'lumpy' the breast tissue. The problem is that women most at risk of breast cancer are far more likely to have dense breast tissue, making emerging small tumours very hard to spot.

Doctors recommend women over 40 should have the test annually as early detection provides better rates of cure and can offer the choice of a lumpectomy rather than a full mastectomy. However, each mammogram delivers a high dose of radiation – up to 1,000 times that of a normal X-ray – and there is much debate as to whether the mammograms themselves do more harm than good.

A two-year study in Denmark, originally published in the Lancet and updated in October 2001 suggests that a number of flaws in the mammography process makes the test 'virtually useless'. This has caused controversy and even anger amongst the medical profession.

The European Breast Cancer conference in March 2004 stated that in dense tissue mammograms were no more effective than 59 per cent. (In soft tissue the maximum figure was 67 per cent.) Dr Van der Horst said that dense tissue was on the increase and made it "harder to pick up tumours ... and may lead to unnecessary biopsies".

Dr Kelly McMasters, a surgical oncologist at the University of Louisville is quite clear that the current technology is still showing results and is a lot better than examining yourself. 'The problem with palpation is that when a tumour is big enough to feel it's often spread already to the lymph nodes. This makes it more likely to be fatal'.

The jury is out, and women should make absolutely sure they understand all the risks, and whether they will feel confident in the results.

They must also be clear that they understand the results. 50 per cent of the 'findings' of mammograms are in fact DCIS, calciferous particles in the ducts. At least 80 per cent never lead to a cancer, and these deposits at worst are only pre-cancerous (UCLA, March 2004).

Testicular self-examination
It is not hard to examine the testes. Testicular cancer is most common in the 15-40 age group. The test should be carried out monthly after a warm shower, by rolling each testicle slowly and gently between the thumb and fingers. Any small lump or hard object should be examined by a doctor. Other signs to watch for are dull aches in the testicle, groin or abdomen. This is a highly curable disease especially if caught early.

Sigmoidoscopy

A sigmoidoscope is a narrow tube with a light at the end. Inserted in the rectum it can find polyps and tumours in the lower colon. By contrast a colonoscopy is a longer tube and looks further in to the colon. A newer system called flexible sigmoidoscopy, aims to detect precancerous growths using a miniature camera inserted into the bowel.

The UK Health Minister announced at a national cancer conference that he is intending to introduce a national bowel cancer screening programme for everybody over the age of 50, and is awaiting final results from a Cancer Research UK study.

Two approaches to screening are under consideration, one of which involves testing faeces for early signs of cancer, while the other uses sigmoidoscopy to detect the pre-cancerous growths.

Pap smear

Created by Dr Papaniculaou in the 1940s it has been a major contributor to the lowered rates of **cervical cancer** since that time. The test can detect both pre-cancerous and cancerous cells in the cervix.

The test involves inserting a speculum into the vagina so the cervix can be clearly seen. Sample cells are then taken from the outer part of the cervix using a spatula and using a brush from the inner part. A pelvic examination is also conducted at the same time. An annual smear is recommended after the commencement of sexual activity.

In July 2004 Professor Julian Peto at Cancer Research UK estimated that smear testing was saving 5,000 lives per year in the UK, as up to half the young women in Britain were infected with a high risk strain of HPV by the time they were 30 years old.

Tumour markers

A number of factors are to be found in the blood each indicating the presence of a cancer. Measuring their presence and level can be helpful not just to indicate the cancer but to monitor the effectiveness of treatments.

PSA test

If you are 50 years or over and living in the West there is a very

143

good chance you will have an enlarged non-malignant **prostate** (termed benign prostatic hyperplasia). This carries with it certain symptoms, which are virtually identical to those of prostate cancer.

The UK charity, The Prostate Cancer Charity, defines them as:

- Difficulty or pain when passing urine
- The need to pass urine more often
- Broken sleep due to the need to pass urine
- Waiting for long periods before the urine flows
- The feeling that the bladder has not completely emptied.

With prostate cancer you may also suffer from blood in the urine, and/or lower back pain and/or dribbling. But be aware that many of the above symptoms can be caused by other factors e.g. bacterial infection.

Your doctor can simply feel if you have an enlarged prostate (a digital rectal examination). If he finds such an enlargement he will probably send you for a PSA test (prostate-specific antigen). This measures a specific protein in a man's blood, the level of which was thought to correlate with prostate cancer.

However, this test has been found to be flawed. In one research study, factors found in the blood from high dairy consumption, vigorous exercise, or riding a bicycle in the previous 24 hours increased PSA levels.

Indeed, the test does not seem to fully distinguish between enlarged malignant prostates and non-malignant ones, and one USA report concluded that as many as two thirds of those testing positive, probably are not! Never just have a single test, but three to six across a two month period.

CA125
CA125 levels can be used to detect ovarian cancer at an early stage. However although a number of other cancers can increase the level of CA125, so too can a number of benign conditions like endometriosis, fibroids and even pregnancy. For this reason the test is seen as flawed.

Pyruvate kinase
The majority of solid tumour cancers over-express this enzyme

and this can aid detection. Pyruvate kinase testing in the blood is used as a diagnostic by a number of specialist clinics and seems to be pretty accurate. Unfortunately the majority of GP's and oncologists neither perform the test, nor are qualified to read the results.

Others

There are several current tests to ascertain whether a cancer is present. No one is particularly decisive but together they can give a reasonably accurate picture of events:

Interleukin and Interferon: can both show immune response levels

CA15-3 : breast cancer

CA19-9 : oesophageal, bile duct and pancreas

CEA   : oesophageal, lung, bile, colon, pancreas and bladder. However as before, no one of these is perfect and a complex picture has to be studied.

Now scientists from the Federal Drug Agency (FDA) and National Cancer Institute (NCI) in the USA have reported on another as yet unnamed protein test taking just 30 minutes and using a small sample of patient's blood. Although the authors caution that more work is needed to understand the sensitivity of the test, the initial tests identified 50 out of 50 cancer, and 63 out of 66 non-cancer samples.

There is no doubt accurate protein tests could be of significant benefit. For example, currently more than 80 per cent of ovarian cancer patients are diagnosed at a late clinical stage and have a less than 20 per cent chance of five-year survival. In contrast early diagnosis results in 95 per cent survival over the same period making the possibility of protein tests a truly exciting development.

For more information use: www.cancer.gov/newscenter.

(ii) Some examples of new methods being developed

The camera you swallow

The M2A is a camera the size of a vitamin pill and developed by the US firm Given Imaging. When swallowed this battery powered device generates 57,000 images as it passes through the stomach and through the intestine. To date it has been used at the Royal Hallamshire Hospital to discover the causes of intestinal bleeding, but its potential to study polyps, tumours and bowel cancer is enormous. At £300 a time it is the ultimate disposable camera!

Testicular scanner on trial
The world's largest trial to see if a new scanner can improve treatment for testicular cancer patients has been launched by Cancer Research UK.

Scientists funded by the charity will use a sophisticated Positron Emission Tomography (PET) scan to search for early signs of cancer spread in order to identify those at risk of relapse after surgery.

The PET scanner relies on differences in the way tumour cells and normal tissue metabolise glucose to hunt down the active tumour tissue.

New prostate tests
Scientists now believe they have a way to identify **prostate** cancers, which are aggressive and those that are not. To date measurement has always looked at the stage, or spread, of the cancer but there has been little evidence on the grade, or how rapidly the cancer is growing. The problem is that some men with small, yet rapidly growing cancers have not been spotted in time. Now scientists can test the tumours of newly diagnosed patients to discover how aggressive the cancer is. The test involves measuring the amount of an enzyme present in the blood. This enzyme is only produced by cancer cells.

A trial, reported in the scientific journal *Cancer* in September 2002, involved 105 prostate surgery samples. The test is probably applicable to **breast** and **colon** cancers as well.

(iii) Genetic testing
An example:
Women can now be screened for the presence of faulty BRCA1 and BRCA2 genes. Genes are little messages sitting on the ball of string which is your DNA. These are dubbed erroneously the 'breast cancer genes' as, in the 6–7 per cent of women who have

these genes, breast cancer is a high risk. In fact BRCA1 is connected with the immune system and BRCA2 with DNA repair. Both genes have also been linked to a percentage of prostate cancers whilst other, similar genes have been identified for colon and other cancer risks.

The hope is that drugs can be developed to switch off these genes, if their mechanism of cause can be accurately determined. For the time being women identified as having these genes are offered preventative mastectomies or the drug Tamoxifen. This drug has been shown to have benefits, but also it is itself classified as a carcinogen by the World Health Organisation, as it has definite cancer causing risks.

It is appropriate that women with these genes are not influenced by scare mongering, but do take sensible lifestyle and dietary precautions. Recent research covered in **icon** has shown that 50 years ago less than 40 per cent of people with these faulty genes developed cancer but now this figure is approaching 75 per cent. Clearly then, modern diet and lifestyle factors are playing a significant role and people (women and men) with any of these genes could do a lot worse than follow some of the recommendations in this book, to build themselves their own microclimate of health.

SECTION III

You are more than just a machine

'Mind over matter'

Introduction

I walked out of my hotel in the middle of China early one cold December morning and saw a fascinating sight. About 80 Chinese, the youngest in their 60s, all fully clothed and complete with jackets and hats to brave the weather, were standing practising t'ai chi in rows in a dusty square. Slow movements as graceful as a thick coat would allow. No one broke sweat and certainly no one experienced 'the burn'.

As we went off to the medical centre on our two hour journey by bus, we saw perhaps just 50 cars or lorries but literally thousands of people of all ages on their bicycles.

At the medical centre the doctor looked at my eyes, tongue and ears. He told me I had a colon problem and gave me herbs. In London the same diagnosis had required three specialists, X-rays and a barium meal.

I was taken for a massage, offered acupuncture and shown how this was used in place of anaesthetic in operations. The doctor was in fact very open-minded and objective about Western medicine and claimed he would certainly use it if it offered better results.

China had a terrible infant mortality record in the past but this is improving rapidly. According to my Chinese doctor, remove infant mortality from the life expectancy figures and the Chinese would expect to live longer than Europeans or Americans. What will we do if one day those figures are clearly borne out in the West? Will our medical authorities be as open-minded or keen to learn?

Q27. How are we really doing on cancer prevention and cure?

Modern medicine undeniably has helped us to live longer, wiping out diseases and infections that used to kill. But its conquests are becoming less and less effective as the tide of illness mounts.

The average life expectancy of an American in 1900 was 48. By 1920 it was 57 and by 1990 any new baby could expect to live to 75. Great strides.

However, if you take out infant mortality from the figures and ask how long if you were 50 would you expect to live, in 1920, he or she could expect to live to 74; and by 1990 to 78. This 7–8 per cent improvement is no mean achievement but far less than many people would suppose across a 70 year period, considering all the money that has been poured into research, medicines, and the health services.

Since 1980 this age-adjusted life expectancy figure has hardly increased at all.

The five-year survival rates for people with cancer in the USA improved by about 10 per cent between 1974 and 1990, going from 49 per cent to 54 per cent. However since 1990 this figure has remained virtually static. In England, five-year survival rates have improved by just 12 per cent in the last 30 years (National Audit Office).

Statistically, early detection has not increased cure rates and, with a couple of very notable exceptions (e.g. child leukaemia), a large number of current treatments do not seem to prolong over-all life. Perhaps this is because, whilst science advances, other factors like diet, stress and health risks are acting in the opposite direction. Perhaps, dare I suggest(?), the emphasis on the curative route the medical profession is taking, with its increasing focus on just surgery, radiotherapy and chemotherapy, is fatally flawed.

Take cancer death ages and there is little difference over time, yet the population as a whole is ageing. Indeed, the average age of death from cancer has hardly changed in 15 years. Part of the reason for this is that more younger people are contracting it.

More people now contract cancer. In the USA in 2001 there

were 1.3 million new cases of cancer and 550,000 deaths. These figures have increased by 60 per cent since 1950. New cases are estimated to exceed 1.6 million by 2005.

In a survey of industrialised nations (including USA, Europe, and Japan) non-smoking related cancers account for 78 per cent of this growth, with a growth in prostate cancer of 200 per cent, breast cancer of 64 per cent, and child cancers of 35 per cent. Although Japan has cancer rates considerably lower than in the West, breast cancer has risen by 100 per cent in the same period.

In the UK there were around 267,000 new cases of cancer in the year 2003. Mortality levels were:

Lung cancer	34,250
Large bowel cancer	16,000
Breast cancer	13,500
Prostate cancer	9,500
Stomach cancer	7,000
Oesophageal cancer	7,000

Also, one has to be careful of exactly how the figures are presented. One oncologist told me that breast cancer sufferers had an 85 per cent chance of surviving five years and published data claims that around 80 per cent of cases are successfully treated. However a simple piece of maths shows that last year there were 39,500 new cases in the UK. In the same year 13,500 women died from it, a figure of 35 per cent of the new cases, indicating a 65 per cent long-term survival rate. Obviously some of these are outside the five year period but it portrays a truer figure for overall survival rates. But the truth is that there are only a few cancers that can be genuinely totally cured despite the billions of pounds spent and the quality of the people involved.

Having read this, if you have cancer, I urge you not to fret. As I keep saying, these are figures for the 'average' person and this book will help you become much better than the average person in beating cancer. Secondly, as we will cover later, you can live a happy, long and fulfilled life even if some cancer cells remain. Controlling your cancer, for example with a strong immune system, is a very sensible and realistic route to follow.

There are a couple of other points worth noting. Advertising claims by a leading charity in the UK that the words 'all clear' are being heard more and more these days are sadly more due to the increased level of cancer rather than great strides in the, so called, cure rate. As shown above the official Government statistics show only a 12 per cent improvement in 30 years. Hardly a record to be shouting about on TV screens or posters!

In fact in October 2003, in Breast Cancer Awareness Month, the charity reported that the disease of cancer was at record levels. In 2004 a team of UK cancer experts, co-ordinated by the charity MacMillan Cancer Relief, predicted that the number of cancer cases in Britain would treble over the next 20 years, 'decimating the National Health Service' unless urgent action was taken.

In the Eurocare-3 study in 2003 the poor record of treatment in the UK is highlighted. With Sweden and France each having five-year survival rates of over 80 per cent (82.6 and 81.5 respectively) in England the figure is 73.6 per cent, which is below the European average of 76.1 per cent and just above Latvia and Estonia. For prostate cancer our five-year survival rates are even more adrift at 53.8 per cent compared with a European average of 65.4 per cent, and countries like Austria (83.6 per cent), Germany (75.9 per cent) and France (75.2 per cent). Why do our charities and cancer agencies so over claim their success in the UK? Why is there so much arrogance and complacency within the UK medical system about cancer?

Maybe treatments other than surgery, chemotherapy and radiotherapy are needed to improve rates? In Germany, for example, doctors have to offer alternative treatments if their first ideas fail; many are also qualified homeopaths; many use Vega testing. In Austria, herbs are widely used.

Meanwhile we seem determined to ape the drugs and the treatments of the USA, a country the WHO has just listed as number 37 in the world in terms of 'health of the population'!

The current Genome Project work may have enormous potential. Scientists have mapped your complete DNA 'string', showing which parts correspond to your eyes, ears and legs; and also showing little pieces of code that determine cancers in your body. Scientists are currently working on how to switch off these pieces

155

of code. However, whether they will be able to 'play' with your genes without causing extra problems in the body remains to be seen.

Different countries spend vastly different amounts on cancer cure. For example, the spending in 2000 on cancer therapy drugs per capita was:-

USA	$10.86
Germany	$8.74
Italy	$5.33
UK	$1.33

Sadly against all this activity little focus is placed on **prevention**.

As we saw in Section I, the Western world's weight of money from government, charities and drug companies pouring into cancer cures is quite incredible. Without wishing to seem cynical, this is because of several factors, none of which has much to do with the health of the nation. Hardly a day passes without a story in the national press about trials of a new wonder drug. It's good copy and it shows that people are trying. Charities want more money to explore cancers and look for cures so they can show successes and results. Governments want to be seen to be supporting a health service that currently has sick patients sitting in long queues. Drug companies have a symbiotic relationship with doctors and governments to do their best to supply the cures, notwithstanding the profits they will make.

The rising rates of cancer have come about slowly across a 50 year or more period and reversing this trend could be expected to take a similar period, even if it were possible. Since most company bosses, presidents and prime ministers don't last much more than 50 months, this doesn't come too high on their agendas. And anyway, given the high levels of non-smoking related cancers and their diversity, how could you afford the structures necessary to monitor all possible toxins and their effects in areas such as household or cosmetic or toiletry products or industrial waste and nuclear power stations or food crops and water supplies, or magnetic fields from aerials and power lines? Even where quite good controls already exist, how would you start scientifically to monitor and improve the interaction of it all?

These are the challenges facing us all. Clearly every thinking person who cares about the world they are passing on to the next generation ought to be making their voice heard and the Government, schools and the media all have a role to play, but then so does every parent in the Western world doing the cooking or buying the household products. Meanwhile all we can try to do is to create our own little micro-environments as best we can. We all need to understand the carcinogens that attack us and the lifestyle elements that destroy us. We can at least take some sensible steps in the areas open to our own control. And, if the worst happens and we succumb to cancer, we need to realise that there are diet, medical, lifestyle and complementary approaches outside our standard Western medical thinking that definitely can help us all.

As Lily Tomlin once said, '*We're all in this together ... On our own!*'

Q28. Is it possible that 'scientific cancer cures' are not addressing the real problem?

Cancer is systemic. Its effects may be noticed all over the body. For example, if you take a sample of blood from someone with a brain tumour (even though the actual tumour never produces secondaries in other parts of the body) you will still see two things:

- The white cells are static, indicating an impaired immune system; and people with lowered immune systems, according to US research, get more cancers. Love your immune system!
- The red cells will be clumped indicating poor oxygen levels, a condition favoured by cancer cells. Keep oxygen in your blood system!

This is true whether the original cancer is in the head or the toe, the breast or the prostate.

Clearly the only way to 'eliminate' a problem that runs throughout the body is to provide a total body solution. It is doubtful that a localised treatment like surgery or radiotherapy could ever succeed on its own; and chemotherapy would only succeed if it destroyed all the contributing factors, and all the cancer and precancer cells.

You, your body, your attitude and your 'total personal programme' have to 'make up the difference'.

There is a celebrated doctor and health guru called Deepak Chopra who runs a clinic called the Chopra Centre for Well Being in La Costa, California. He believes fervently that you can not only stop the ravages of ageing and disease but with effort and care you can actually reverse them.

He, like a lot of people who have studied Eastern medicine, believes that the mind, body and soul are inexorably linked. Poor thoughts in the mind or depression take their toll on bodily performance. This is not some cranky thinking but now well established medically.

Every cell in your body is made up of atoms, which in turn are merely particles spinning round other particles in electromagnetic fields largely composed of air. Everyday your body takes in new atoms and expels others so that you completely change all the cells, and all the atoms, in your body every few weeks. Why should it not be possible to kick out a cancer if you could work out what caused it and moreover what exactly was sustaining it? If your diet or lifestyle gave you the cancer originally, why would it not be possible to change them both and return your body to its original healthy state?

The body must be seen as far, far more than the sum of the mechanical parts, and ultimately it will be totally understood that every single one of us has within us the ability to heal and repair a damaged part.

We've all heard stories of love healing, or the power of positive thinking overcoming disease, or even the power of prayer. But then our body is a summation of all these atoms in their magnetic fields within one enormous magnetic field, the universe. Of course there could be an interaction between two beings, or between your mind and the atoms in your liver; or between your energetic being and the energy of the universe.

It is most certainly the case that modern medicine will not succeed in increasing cancer cure rates unless it takes a broader perspective and realises that it has to treat the total patient, rather than merely the cancer.

Now you may consider all this alternative stuff is for cranks, so let's look at a few random facts about the total you, even if indeed they do seem a little strange sometimes.

- More of the world believes in and uses complementary medicine than uses modern 'orthodox' Western medicine. A better name for such medicine would be traditional, natural healing. In fact at least twice as many people in the world use diet and natural healing as use modern drug-based medicine. In the UK,

159

40 per cent of all cancer patients have at least one form of complementary therapy (Macmillan).

- One American study stated that with certain cancers an individual was two to three times more likely to achieve a cure through diet and supplements than through radiotherapy and chemotherapy combined. Q48 will tell you of the Gonzalez success with just such a diet and supplement programme over conventional chemotherapy.

- Certain cancers are almost non-existent in China and south east Asia; is this despite their diets, or because of them? Take a Chinese person to New York and they are statistically just as likely to develop a cancer as the native New Yorker.

- Animals like bears and gorillas never get cancer in the wild. Keeping them in zoos with unnatural diets and stressful surroundings causes seven out of 10 to get cancer.

- Researchers have found that women who have three orgasms a week have higher levels of immunoglobin A and boost their immune systems by up to 30 per cent! Apparently every time women reach orgasm their bodies produce more T-lymphocytes to better resist infection and fight cancer. Good sex also produces growth hormone and releases endorphins, so-called happy hormones that neutralise anxiety and stress hormones in the body. If that wasn't enough girls, in a study of women with breast cancer those who had regular orgasms recovered faster than those who didn't.

- Reiki, or hands on healing, has so powerful an effect on the chakras (spiritual centres in the body) that it cannot be used whilst someone is having radiotherapy or chemotherapy because its healing power reduces their effectiveness.

- Chinese doctors do not like to poison the immune system of their patients with anaesthetics. They operate using acupuncture leaving the patient with no after-effects at the end of the surgery and the strongest possible immune system to fight the underlying illness.

- Yoga and meditation have been proven to boost the immune system by around 30 per cent.

- One study showed that people with a God or people with religious beliefs, like for like, live on average seven years longer

160

than the norm. Another showed that people who attend church regularly live on average seven years longer than those who don't. At Dukes in Carolina, doctors have recently noticed that those sufferers who believe in a God do indeed survive longer, and they are about to conduct specific research into this finding.

All of the above indicate that there are healing factors well beyond those normally considered by Western medicine. I am not saying use alternative medicine instead of radiotherapy. By and large radiotherapy does knock back cancers. The question is, can we use broader based therapies beyond those of Western science to help improve rates for cancer cure or to prevent cancer in the first place? And the answer is, undoubtedly, YES!

Q29. What other factors can affect my general health and well-being?

In the West, orthodox medicine envisages the body as a machine where we are now able to remove a part such as a heart or kidney that is not functioning properly and replace it. The case for cloning that is argued in the media and by governments, is that scientists could end up with a perfect set of spare parts for each of us if and when something breaks down.

What if we were more than a complex set of machine parts? What if each of our mechanical parts was imbued with an over-riding system that was uniquely ours? What if this over-riding system was more powerful in terms of our health than the mechanical part?

Each of us has a body energy system unique to us.

There are three models of this. One from China that spread throughout the Far East, one that had its origin in India and a third developed relatively recently in the West.

The Western version is very similar to the Indian model. Around your body there are seven layers of energy fields that each have their own frequency, colour, density and fluidity and together form your aura. We know they exist!

A Russian, Kirlian, developed a method of photographing this aura 30 or so years ago. American scientists have done a lot of work on this in recent years measuring it, weighing it and study-ing, in particular, how two people might communicate between their auras. The frequency of the energy fields and the colours they emit change with the mood of the individual, for example, if they are angry or being untruthful, and with their health.

The seven layers each come from one of seven points on your body, each being a spinning vortex of energy called a chakra, down the centre line of your body.

The first layer is linked to your first chakra at the base of your spine, the second to your sacrum, the third to your solar plexus, the fourth to your heart, the fifth to your throat, the sixth to your forehead and the seventh to your crown. Each also links to an organ in the endocrine system e.g. the sixth to the pineal gland. The first three chakras are concerned with elements of your physical being like practicality or emotion, the fourth is connected to the heart and associated with love, whilst the outermost, highest three layers are linked to the spiritual plane.

You can have auric pictures taken of your fingertips which not only show aura lines radiating out from them, but the nerve endings connected (depending upon the finger and the position) to each of the body's organs. If there are toxins in the organ, the colour of the auric lines actually changes and can be used for diagnosis. I know, I've seen mine and the diagnosis was spot on!

When you lose someone you love dearly, poets would like us to believe you suffer a broken heart. But actually it is the chakra of emotion that suffers, giving you a painful sensation not in the heart region but in the solar plexus at the top of the stomach.

Our energy layers interact with those of other people just as the magnetic fields interacted when we saw experiments with magnets and iron filings at school. And we know that some people make us happy to be with them, while others simply drain our energy.

Our energy levels interact with our environment. A bird singing may calm us, a warm bath will relax us (it temporarily reduces our auric field), the sound of a glass window pane breaking at four in the morning may frighten us, a storm may stress us. American scientists have studied the basis of these energy systems and proven that you have channels, which take the energy fields inside the body to the internal organs. The blocking of channels can lead to illness, and acupuncture works by unblocking these channels.

Illness is believed to start with your energy flow being weakened or disrupted. In other words your energy system becomes unbalanced and gets ill first.

Dr Richard Gerber in his book *Vibrational Medicine* said, *'From an energetic standpoint, the human body when weakened oscillates at a different and less harmonious frequency than when healthy. If the same individual is supplied with a dose of the needed energetic frequency it allows the cellular bioenergetic systems to resonate in the proper vibrational mode, thereby throwing off the illness'*.

163

Since your chakras link to:

- The practicalities of your life
- Your emotions
- Love (and your relationship with others)
- Your spiritual relationship with the universe.

All these things can, and do, make you ill. There are some people who are naturally full of energy. They seem to radiate it, whilst others are depressed and lifeless.

And so we have a picture building up, that your energy system is linked to your brain and your emotions, to your endocrine system and your hormones, to your nervous system and to your internal organs. And to the universe around each of us.

Clearly, then, all of us who want to prevent or cure a cancer need to be aware of our own body energy and to do everything in our power to keep it flowing strongly and smoothly, ensuring that it is in balance and cleansed. All of us should on a regular basis see expert cranial osteopaths, acupuncturists, masseurs, reflexologists, reiki masters, homeopaths, aromatherapists; take your pick

Everybody should think of taking up yoga, t'ai chi or some other exercise that aims to regulate and improve the flow of energy in their bodies as a regular weekly habit. But be careful, you also just might enjoy it!

Q30. How important is my mental attitude?

Crucial.
Why is it that two patients with same affliction react so differently? One will take himself off to bed, while the other runs, plays sport, goes out and laughs it off.

Everybody stamps their condition with their own unique personality.

Death rates from cancer are higher among people in psychological distress and lower in people with a stronger sense of self-worth and self-purpose. Fact. Yet mechanically these people are the same. No wonder a doctor's work is so difficult.

Fear-motivated behaviour, guilt, depression, people who feel imperfect, inadequate, people who dwell in the past, who strive to be something they are not, people who judge others and themselves all the time, these people get ill.

In fact, people used to treating cancer patients describe a typical cancer sufferer as someone who 'tends to be a nice person, who wants to please and be liked. These people do not hold themselves in very high esteem and feel the cancer is somehow what they deserve'. The truth about these people is that with emotional scars and a feeling of always atoning for their sins or inadequacies, they don't nurture themselves enough, they don't respect themselves enough and they don't value themselves enough.

Cancer patients don't just need to change their physical lifestyle and diet, they need to change their mental attitude too.

Relax, be content with yourself, live in neither the past nor the future but here and now, don't apologise or feel guilty, be happy, have fun, love life, love yourself, think nice things, don't be habitually critical. Most importantly realise that you have strengths and skills, that you are a 'loved' person who deserves the best in life and has the ability deep inside you to be special.

'Our deepest fear is not that we are inadequate. Our deepest fear is that we are powerful beyond measure. It is our light, not our darkness, that most frightens us. We ask ourselves: "Who am

I to be brilliant, gorgeous, talented, fabulous?" Actually, who are you not to be? You are a child of God. Your playing small doesn't serve the world'. This was written by a man with every reason to be depressed and inadequate after years of imprisonment often fearing for his life and that he might never be free; Nelson Mandela.

In his book *The Road Less Travelled*, Scott Peck tells us to equate, 'Time with value with love'. If you love a baby you value it and you want to spend time with it. So too with yourself. Everyone must find time to love themselves and to show themselves that they value their life and being in good health. Time to shop properly for fresh produce or to cook nutritious foods, time to have a Thai massage, time to take exercise, time to be calm.

Henry Kissinger once said, *'Next week there can't be any crisis; my schedule is already full.'* And that's the world we live in.

Stress, crises, unhappiness, fear of inadequacy, fear of failure are just some of the negative forces at work in our minds. Unfortunately the very people who have emotional problems are most prone to smoke and drink and not to look after themselves. This is less because of the pressure of work and practicalities, and more because of their emotional needs. If you can work on your emotional needs and fears, and strengthen your sense of purpose you will respect yourself more. Surely smoking heavily or pouring excess alcohol down your throat is a sign that you have little respect for yourself or your body.

Time magazine (20 January 2003) carried a 40 page special entitled 'How your mind can beat your body'. This collected the latest information from a huge number of sources.

It showed how, by using Positron-Emission Tomography or Functional Magnetic Resonance, pictures of the brain could be taken linking brain activity with diseases in different parts of the body. When you have a cancer in a certain part of your body, a shadow is observed on the part of the brain corresponding to that part of the body.

The brain is just one of many body organs and exhibits the same biochemistry as all the other organs. When the brain is depressed the biochemical activity of the cells in the brain exhibits certain characteristics. These are then communicated to the heart, lungs or breast and those cells will mirror the same biochemistry. Brain chemicals such as serotinin, for example, circulate throughout the body.

It is thus no surprise that people who are depressed have higher rates of heart disease and cancer. In November 2002 top experts in America met in Washington to discuss the evidence linking depression with disease. Depression is known to alter the structure of the blood making blood cells less likely to clump together. They carry less oxygen and this helps oxygen-hating cancer thrive, and they indirectly increase inflammation around the arteries.

Twenty per cent of diabetic women have depression, and depression makes the body less responsive to insulin. Insulin plays a role in cancer too. Depression affects cortisol levels and like insulin this stimulates localised bad eicosanoid production.

Stress results in the release of a flood of hormones in the body which affect nervous responses, organs and cellular biochemistry. Even low level stress is linked with low levels of circulating glucocorticoids, which in turn lead to a greatly weakened immune system.

Naturopathy and PNEI

Naturopathy is an ancient system of healing, which encourages building immunity naturally by viewing the individual as an integral part of nature's big picture.

Conventional medicine has recently overlapped with naturopathy through the study of Psycho-Neuro-Endocrino-Immunology or PNEI

Put simply: our feelings, emotions and thoughts are fundamentally connected to the working of our bodies.

PNEI is founded on two important principles:

- That in a hostile and toxic environment two people can differ completely in their susceptibility to illness. This is due, in naturopathic terms, to a personal and individual immunity; an inner profile.
- That there is a clear link between different emotions and both the nervous and endocrine system. Substances are then secreted, which actually affect receptor points on the cellular membrane

(probably through the eicosanoid system). So biochemically a stressful situation in your workplace 'stresses' your cells. A depressing meeting affects your mood and depresses your cells. A person who feels worthless has 'worthless' cells.

Both a healthy outer energy system and a strong inner profile provide immunity. But equally, a weakened energy system, or stressful emotional situations weaken your immunity. Not surprisingly people in continuous depressed states have been shown to have immune systems 30 per cent weaker than the norm.

Your mind is linked to your body energy. It is linked to your hormones and your nervous system and, through receptors, to your cells, and thus your cellular biochemistry.

So what can any of us do?

Firstly, as I have said, take time for yourself. Be idle, be calm, relax, meditate, take a massage, learn yoga. It is not a sin to do nothing. As Robert Louis Stevenson said, 'To be idle requires a strong sense of personal identity.'

Secondly, as any good life coach will tell you, achieving a better life is not always about setting goals and striving. There is more often the need to remove from your life those things or people that limit you, or hold you back, or cause you most stress and pain.

There are too many people in this world who try to make you feel guilty or smaller or subservient. This is because they cannot generate their own vital energy and need to draw it from others. If you have a colleague, friend or even partner who does this, you must recognise that ultimately it may make you ill, and act accordingly. Start by analysing yourself. What causes you hurt, distress or pain; which people criticise you unfairly or make you feel guilty? Cut these things and these people out of your life for your health's sake. This is the first step to rebuilding your self-esteem.

It is a well studied fact that all animals and people are either providers or takers of energy. By and large children and animals are takers of energy. Large dogs and horses are providers of energy, adult humans can be either providers or takers depending upon their emotional background and stability.

168

Surround yourself with a real support group. Optimists, positive thinkers, happy people, people with their own energy, vitality and ideas. Avoid the pessimists, the critics and the moaners.

Where you cannot remove extreme emotional stress after, say, the loss of a close family member, you have to put it in the context of your own life and try to be positive about it. Counselling or visualisation, especially if you are seriously ill, may well be a good idea.

To best avoid illness you must have a strong sense of purpose about your own life. This is often quite weak in cancer sufferers, many of whom like spend more time trying to please those around them, or doing things to impress and gain plaudits rather than seeking things that make them happy themselves. Eventually, of course, these people end up not being true to themselves.

To be at your healthiest you need to have:

- An honest understanding of your own strengths and weaknesses
- An honest understanding of your own identity, your likes and dislikes
- A sense of purpose which genuinely reflects the above and is yours and not modified by other people's desires for you.

Be at peace with yourself. You have wonderful strengths so start to recognise them and appreciate yourself. Be positive in all your beliefs. Develop the 'I can do it' mentality. As Henry Ford said, *'Whether you think you can or you think you cannot, you are usually right!'* Be in no doubt that you are physically the summation of how you feel about yourself.

Naturopathy is at the basis of most alternative health treatments. It holds a number of fundamental tenets:

- Health is psycho-physiological. The distinction between mind and body is artificial. The more physical the symptom, the more psychologically accented needs to be the treatment.
- Health is nutrition. You are what you eat. If your crops failed to grow you would look to their nutrients, from soil to rainfall. So too with your body.
- Health is movement. Movement and posture increase natural

energy flow, improve circulation and the health of the internal organs, dissipate nervous energy and toxins.

- Health is concerned with the quality of life not merely the duration.

Naturopathy holds a simple belief that the body has the power to heal itself. When your body is in pain your tears show evidence of the endocrine system starting the healing process. Modern medicine overrides this, giving counter-action medicines such as antibiotics, anti-inflammatories and antidepressants. This approach, called allopathy, is directed against the signs or symptoms of the disease. It is not intended to find the root cause, the underlying problem, merely to cover up the symptoms in the hope that that is enough.

But if you want to prevent cancer it is imperative you work on your underlying health.

Cancer is the symptom of another illness; one which may have started even now to overtake your greater body and one you must address if you really want to beat it.

All of this can be summarised as follows:

A healthy body starts with a happy attitude, a sense of purpose, and a total feeling of self worth and value. This feeling in itself directly stimulates the nervous and endocrine systems, making your immune system and your cellular biochemistry stronger. This will in turn make you happier and lead you to value yourself more, for example, in your approach to your life, friends and work or in taking exercise, in taking time for yourself, in choosing what you should or shouldn't eat. This in turn further stimulates the immune system and builds your body energy. This is the way to beat cancer, and indeed all illness.

Q31. How can I revitalise my energy?

In Eastern philosophies energy systems are seen as a reflection of the universe, and are influenced by diet, climate and environment plus mental and spiritual attitudes.

Chi (in China), ki (in Japan) and prana (in India) are words for energy. Hence rei ki is Universal Energy.

Chi (also known as qi) is the Chinese term for 'vital energy' and enters the body through the air we breathe and the food we eat. Poor, unclean air and poor breathing habits such as shallow breathing both result in imbalance and thus illness.

Chi flows through the body along a network of channels, the meridians. There are 12 major ones, most linking to an organ in the body. Each meridian has a channel on either side of the body. Yang energy comes from the sun and flows down the body, yin comes from the earth and flows up the body.

If a person is unhealthy the energy flow is uneven, disturbed or even blocked. We all know that the wrist has a pulse for the blood system. At almost the same point each wrist has three pulse points for energy, each corresponding to certain organs, so that six organs in total are represented.

Most of the effective methods of revitalising energy come from Eastern philosophies. Here are some examples:

Qigong

Over 60 million Chinese use qigong which develops a body's energy in four ways – breathing, movement, body stance or posture and meditation. Exercise, breathing and posture develop the body's energy and flow whilst specific exercises can be used to unblock meridians

T'ai chi

Millions of people practise t'ai chi each morning. Graceful, physical movements and breathing combine with balance to improve the circulation, open up the lymph systems and the flow of vital energy, in turn stimulating the immune system. T'ai chi exercises stem from qigong, with the emphasis being on the mind, relaxation and internal energy rather than external energy development. As well as being a beneficial set of exercises, tai chi also has martial applications and can be an effective form of self-defence.

Reiki

Reiki is a form of 'hands on' healing where a reiki master imparts universal energy into your chakras; he or she is merely a conduit for that energy. In traditional Japanese medicine ki 'lives' about one inch below the navel and it is here all the energy for the body's support systems finds its roots. The reiki master's hands will often appear very hot (you lie down fully clothed) and you may 'see' flashes of coloured lights even though your eyes are shut. Expert reiki masters are definitely worth a visit and they can recharge you and get your energy flowing again. Reiki masters believe that everyone has the power naturally within them to transmit universal energy and affect another's body energy.

Cranial osteopathy

Cranial osteopaths use the chakras and the line of the backbone to balance energy along the body, often moving energy from one area to another. They will look for blockage which can often be linked to skeletal problems and rebuild the flow and the energy levels where you need it by manipulation of both the skeletal system and energy states. It is well worth seeing a top class cranial osteopath every three months or so for a body energy and skeletal service.

Yoga

Yoga has extraordinary benefits if it is done properly. A great many people know of its ability to increase flexibility but this is just one of its benefits. Yoga aims to affect two important aspects of your body:

- The link between your breathing, your mind and the control of energy into your body
- The opening of the energy channels and chakras to allow maximum flow between them and the internal organs.

Yoga's excellent at releasing and cleansing toxins from the body.

In November 2003, in a study in Seattle, researchers showed that people with high cortisol levels (the stress hormone) could go home and lie down for a week and the level would decline by 5 per cent. But after a first ever session of yoga, another group of patients had cortisol levels that had declined by 25 per cent. And stress is linked to cancer.

Ashtanga yoga is quite an athletic form of yoga perhaps better for younger readers as it involves higher than usual heart rates with exercises that are particularly strong on lymphatic drainage and stretching the body to stimulate the lymphatic system. However all yoga exercises can have a significant effect on unblocking chakras and on the immune system in general.

Pranayama is essentially breathing exercise. There are 72,000 channels or nadis in the body along which energy needs to flow freely for good health. Positions are adopted that link with breath control and these positions help open up channels.

Pranic breathing helps to correct poor breathing habits and encourages the flow of prana purifying the body. We Westerners breathe improperly only using about one third of our lung capacity so that our lungs always carry around stale air and toxins in their lower reaches. Correct breathing comes from correct posture, and using the abdominal muscles to force the diaphragm up and down. It does not come from chest expansion. Masters of this form of yoga 'breathe' in energy through their crown chakra. The process starts re-energising the root chakra and moves up the body through the seven chakras. When all seven chakras are so energised the body reaches its ultimate state of meditation.

Meditation

For some readers, it may seem hard to believe that meditation can actually re-energise you.

Remember that the energy systems, the mind, your breathing, your endocrine system, your nervous system, your blood and your lymph are all linked. Yogis believe that breathing exercises strengthen the body, clear the mind, maintain inner balance and thus help to prevent illness.

State of mind and breathing patterns are known to be linked, for instance, an agitated mind can result in rapid, shallow breathing.

By focusing attention on our breathing it can be gradually slowed and made deeper. This has a calming effect on the whole body and brain. Research has shown that the vibrational frequency of the brain waves changes, with different and slower frequency waves appearing during meditation. This in turn affects the endocrine system. Meditation has a profound effect on reducing cortisol levels which in turn lowers the levels of bad eicosanoids and promotes the levels of good ones. Meditation may involve constant chanting of a word or a noise. To stop the mind wandering you may add a constant theme or thought, for example love, as a focus. This in turn causes the release of favourable hormones inside the body.

Research tests on people who participate in yoga and meditation show higher outer energy states, and immune systems up to 30 per cent stronger than normal.

There is some evidence from Australia that meditation alone can lead to some remarkable cases of cancer healing. It certainly reduces blood pressure and resting heart rate.

Massage

Shiatsu, a Japanese form of massage, involves a professional practitioner examining the flow of energy along the meridians and using deep finger pressure at 'acupoints' to stimulate and regulate it. This benefits the lymph and nervous systems. There is a lot of overlap here with acupuncture, and shiatsu is an approved medical therapy in Japan.

Thai massage traces the lymph system in the body and stimulates its free flow. Like shiatsu, Thai massage involves deep, penetrating finger pressure. Lymph drainage is a term you have probably heard. After massage you must drink plenty of water as toxins will be 'turned out' of the lymph system.

Reflexology

The hands and feet are sites of nerve endings connected to all parts of the body. Sadly, a lot of reflexology resembles a nice foot rub. Done properly it can be diagnostic and re-energising as it helps to remove crystals and blockages, and stimulates the nervous system. These crystals are in fact toxins, which due to gravity, fall to the feet rather than being expelled from the body. If crystals are located, they can be massaged, broken up and then more easily expelled from the body, re-energising the corresponding organ and its blood supply. This can be a little painful depending upon the amount of crystals found.

Acupuncture

Acupuncturists gauge the strength of energy flow through the meridians by checking the six pulses in your wrists, each of which corresponds to an organ in your body. Along each meridian lie acupoints and by inserting a fine needle in some of them, blockages can be removed and a strong energy flow re-established to where it is needed. And, yes, you do feel the needles!

During both acupuncture and cranial osteopathy, you may feel tingling sensations as if water is flowing inside you. If you were particularly out of balance before, you may feel light-headed when you stand, something that can happen with reiki as well.

Acupuncture is now recognised as an important treatment by the medical services in both the USA and the UK.

Exercise

This form of re-energising the body is obviously not linked to Eastern philosophy but research evidence is clear. Exercise helps beat cancer.

Exercise strengthens the heart, the blood system, the lymph system and the skeletal structure. It clears toxins from the lungs, the cells and the blood. It releases 'happy' endorphin hormones, which neutralise negative hormones like adrenaline and it has a hundred other benefits. You are an animal – you are supposed to exercise. No other animal in its natural habit sits on chairs or works at computers.

Anybody who has been to China knows they cycle everywhere, so maybe it is not just the high selenium in their diet and dislike of dairy that keeps them cancer free!

However, walking to the station, a round of golf, making the beds or whatever the tabloids say this week does not officially qualify as exercise, that is, according to the UK Government. Their recommendation is as follows: for 20 minutes, three times per week, you need your heart rate to be between 55 per cent and 85 per cent of its theoretical maximum, which is 220 minus your age.

So, for example, a 50 year old has a maximum of 170 and 85 per cent is about 145. Non-stop, 20 minutes. Before that you warm up and afterwards you cool down.

As both a biochemist and a qualified personal trainer, I feel this is inadequate. Your fitness requirement has a need to stimulate the heart, the peripheral blood system and particularly the more passive lymph system. But this needs to be done every day not three times per week for 20 minutes. Indeed US research (**icon** – Cancer Watch) showed that women who took gentle exercise only, but every day, had 18 per cent less breast cancers.

One school of thought says that, through exercise, you should burn about 3,300 calories per week, which represents one and a half days normal calorie intake for a man. This equates to approximately 470 calories per day, which is about an hour on a bicycle each day. This should be even, calm exercise with the body constantly re-hydrated so that toxins can be taken away. You should eat protein within two hours after exercising and, during the whole process, you should be in control and able to talk without pause. This is a long way from the 'burn' of aerobics or an hour on a squash court. In fact extreme exercise, where you are out of breath and dehydrated, releases lots of toxins which the body must then remove from the cells, so beware. It makes far more of a case for t'ai chi than for a Jane Fonda style aerobics blast.

In January 2005 new US Government health guidelines were published. Previously the authorities had been suggesting 30 minutes exercise per day, something all observers of US waistlines know has not worked. Undaunted, officialdom has now decreed that the new recommendation should be 60–90 minutes per day, every day!

Finally, especially as you age, you need to do some resistance training. Lifting weights keeps up bone density avoiding brittle bones, so there is no need for women to take oestrogen in HRT.

Go the gym instead. Lifting weights until they tire you also helps release a little growth hormone about 20 minutes after you finish This will mop up some free radicals and improve muscle tone and posture allowing energy to flow around the body better.

Two words of warning. Firstly, if you are over the age of 40, do not suddenly take up exercise or rekindle your sporting ambitions of 20 years ago. Work yourself back gradually ideally using a one on one expert or within a professional class. Secondly, drink plenty of water and keep yourself hydrated. If you feel dizzy, stop.

It is interesting to note that researchers at Bristol University have found that physical activity could significantly reduce the risk of bowel cancer by between 40 and 50 per cent and can help in the prevention of breast, prostate, lung and endometrial cancer. They are now studying the positive benefits of exercise for those people undergoing cancer treatment.

Indeed, Cancer Research UK sponsored a study by Bristol of all the worldwide research on exercise and cancer and from 54 studies the conclusion was drawn that exercise can prevent a cancer, and exercise can help recovery.

In summary

I hope this very limited summary of ways of cleansing your body and re-energising it, will have stressed the need to regard the body as much more than the sum of the physical parts. And to help you realise that t'ai chi or reflexology are not cranky mystical hocus pocus but can make a significant contribution to your body energy, endocrine and immune systems and therefore to cancer prevention and cancer cure.

There are many more holistic treatments, for example crystal healing, and clinics such as the Bristol Centre, the Hale Clinic or the Breat Cancer Haven in the UK will be able to impart more information. Suitable books and contact numbers are in the appendices.

Q32. Can homeopathy help?

Strictly speaking, homeopathy does not make any claims where cancer is concerned.

One branch of homeopathy, homotoxicology, looks at disease in six phases of which the first three phases have a favourable prognosis while phases four to six are less favourable but certainly not incurable. Cancer is, however, phase six.

In the average homeopathic practice most patients will come during or after orthodox treatment. Homeopathy can help a cancer sufferer in several ways:

- Firstly, homeopathy can help change someone's mental framework, for example, making them feel less suppressed by their surroundings and more positive with more self esteem.
- Secondly, homeopathy can help eradicate any parasites involved and, in certain cases, boost the body's immune system to fight off any virus that may be present. If you have a parasite or a virus, it can be identified by using EAV (electro-acupuncture according to Voll). A machine from Germany, called a Vega machine, can be used painlessly by a qualified homeopath to look for the presence of infection. Nosodes, best described as natural remedies that help stimulate the body's specific defences to that particular toxin, can be prescribed and the parasite or virus successfully eliminated.
- Thirdly, homeopathy can help detoxify and cleanse, antidote certain toxins, support specific organs and lift the overall body energy, or 'life force'.

In certain cases homeopathy can set up a reaction in the body to reinforce its ability to fight a specific cancer. There are specific nosodes to take for a number of cancers. For example, there is a nosode for brain tumours, and a homeopath I know treated herself and successfully beat breast cancer without radiation or chemotherapy.

It can be an aid during surgery, for example, to decrease bruising.

Finally, it can play a huge supporting role when patients are

178

undergoing radio or chemotherapy. By supporting at the physical level, it helps patients withstand the depleting side effects and increases the effectiveness of both treatments.

Apart from its role with parasites and infections, homeopathy is not particularly relevant for prevention, which is felt to be more a role for diet and lifestyle changes. But if you have a cancer, homeopathy can form a part of a holistic approach to treatment, especially in helping the mind.

As with modern medicine you must find a homeopath who has regular and specific experience of your type of cancer. This can be done through the Society of Homeopaths. Be very choosy. You'd only want the best brain surgeon, don't accept less in your homeopath.

Q33. How can I live a longer life?

Celebrate life; celebrate living

People who are in love have stronger immune systems. People who laugh a lot have stronger immune systems. Women who have regular orgasms have stronger immune systems. Smiling, happiness and joy all release certain beneficial hormones inside the body and these affect your nervous system, your lymph, your immune system and your whole well-being.

Positive thoughts, happiness and love radiate. The third and fourth chakras actually extend outwards, and two people who are deeply in love can have joined chakras. Even first encounters across a cocktail party have been observed with extensions of the third, the solar plexus, the emotional chakra!

Shouldn't you try to radiate more good vibrations? Try it and see what comes back your way. Maybe we can only see this through our sixth sense rather than through our eyes, but it still affects all our relationships. 'You only get back what you put in', or 'what goes round comes round,' would be two more common expressions.

J D Salinger once said, *'I am a kind of paranoic in reverse. I suspect people of plotting to make me happy!'* People will extend their energy systems towards you, if you do towards them.

The mention of spirituality in a book often finds people skipping a few pages: 'What has it got to do with me?' In a Western world that has turned its back on churches, the soul and the mere mention of God, it is all a bit too 'heavy' and often makes us feel a little uncomfortable because we have, in truth, dismissed most of it without too much thought.

But you exist as a mass of spinning electrons and you do have three layers of auric energy that connect you to the universe. A universe that itself is made of energy and is interconnected, so your well-being is inexorably linked with that universe and indeed the energy systems of the trees, plants and other animals around you.

Naturopaths do not view death as the end of life but merely as a part of our everyday lives since it occurs daily in our cellular system. Inevitably, though, all our cells die pretty much simultaneously.

However, given a simple Newtonian principle we all learned at school that 'energy can neither be created nor destroyed', what happens to our energy when we die? Officially, death may be when our heart stops, or our brain ceases to function, but hasn't it got something to do with our energy leaving our mechanical being?

One of the reasons for growing your own vegetables and eating them raw is that apart from getting all the vitamins and minerals untainted and undiminished you actually ingest their 'fresh' energy systems. A pea picked fresh is steamed in two minutes because it contains natural sugars. Kept for three days, molecular change has occurred together with a loss of energy and the sugar has turned to starch, requiring 20 minutes of steaming to cook it. **Fresh is not just about vitamins and minerals, it is about structure and energetic atoms.**

Understanding that the universe will nurture you by providing fresh energy, or stimulate or depress you through the interface with other people's energy systems is an aspect of spirituality. In Dukes, in Carolina, the doctors have noticed that two groups of people with cancer live longer. Those who fight, and those who have a God.

There is a strong argument that the higher success rates in cancer treatment in America over Britain are in part due to a determination not to accept the status quo, to demand second opinions and alternative diagnoses. This fighting spirit is in contrast to an often resigned apathy amongst British patients who leave themselves in the hands of their doctor. Having a fighting spirit is not being a 'pain in the arse', it's about being true to yourself.

Having a God is about being at peace with yourself. Several different studies show that people with a God and people who regularly attend church have longer lives, probably because their beliefs allow them the thought that God is supporting them, which results in them having a happier, more positive mental outlook.

In neither case do you have the stress of being something you

181

are not. Being untrue to yourself does not just make you ill, it is something other people can perceive from your aura, and so it negatively influences their relationship with you.

Inside your energy system you have a core; the Chinese talk about meridians, the ancient Egyptians about a merkaba, Christians about your soul, and the Japanese about the centre of ki. Even if you are not religious the appropriateness of the biblical statement, '*What good will it be for a man if he gains the whole world, yet forfeits his soul?*' (Mathew 16:26) seems exceptionally relevant in this modern world.

We live in a world where all manner of modern day sins pull us in the wrong direction, whether they are alcohol, drugs, gorgeous meals, late night parties or over indulgence. Perhaps we have to ensure that we nourish our souls as much as our physical bodies by appreciating the natural world around us a little more. And we should take the time to do this.

Spirituality is about strengthening our total being (and yes ultimately our immune system), cuddling our children, trying to understand the needs of others, performing acts of kindness, being happy, being trustworthy, truthful, sincere, true to ourselves and so on. Kirlian photography has shown that yogis have much larger auras, which are the product of their humble yet generous spiritual lifestyles, not solely of the physical benefits of yoga.

Spirituality is not confined to a link with a greater energy, God and the universe, death and the after life. It is about the life in your days rather than the days in your life. It's about the life inside you. And the life inside you that can protect and cure you from cancer.

SECTION IV

What do I do if I get cancer?

Important

This section includes tips and advice gleaned from a number of expert sources.

However before embarking on any course of action, or refraining from any action, readers are advised to consult with their own expert practitioner.

The following section must only be viewed as suggestion and nothing more. Neither the author or publisher can be held responsible for any actions taken or avoided as a result of information contained here.

Q34. If I get cancer, what should I do?

People say that when they first hear that six-letter word their head spins and so many thoughts rush through their mind that they miss most of what is then said. 'Will I die?' is the most common thought. The answer to this is very likely 'no', but it is about odds. Right from the first moment you must start trying to improve yours.

Doctors talk about five year survival rates; 150 per 1,000 with lung cancer, 850 per 1,000 with breast cancer. But, of course, that is an average. If you are young, don't smoke and do everything in your power to increase your odds your chances will be much better.

Dr Rosy Daniel, formerly head of the Bristol Cancer help Centre often quotes her research that people who build a programme of activities around their doctor's orthodox regime, increase their chances of success by up to 60 per cent.

To this end we have prepared an information book, *Cancer: Your First 15 Steps*, designed to help you build your own personal prescription of complementary treatments. In our opinion a total integrated disease running throughout the body requires a totally integrated treatment and there is no reason why you should not confidently plan yours.

Remember three out of four people on average survive. Don't be average, be better.

- The NHS cancer referal guidelines (agreed in 2000) state that any patient who has a sign or symptom that could be caused by cancer, has to be referred to a specialist within two weeks.
- At the first consultation have someone with you (your 'buddy') and prepare a list of questions to take with you. Take notes, have a tape recorder (ask first but there should be no problem) and let your buddy ask questions too. Agree with the consultant a convenient time for a further question and answer session because you will get home and find that new questions spring to mind, partly because oncologists 'cushion' the answers to questions for fear of upset, and often seem evasive.

- Ask for your medical notes. Since November 1991 you have a right to see all notes and correspondence relating to your case.
- Find out exactly what the plan is for your recovery, what treatment is to be recommended. Ask about likely problems, how success will be assessed (e.g. complete recovery in six months, going back to work), and what chances there are of the cancer recurring.
- Look into other sources of information and help.

- go to our website www.iconmag.co.uk immediately for the widest and most helpful information on all manner of cancers, treatments and therapies.
- contact the Bristol Cancer Help Centre for their dietary advice for your particular cancer, together with advice on other alternative treatments you can start immediately
- phone the Macmillan Cancer Relief's helpline or the Cancer BACUP and ask specifically for the phone number of the help group relating to your particular cancer
- find a friend who is good on the internet and ask them to help you access your cancer type, looking for any drugs recommended so that you and your buddy can keep informed with absolutely up to the minute information
- go to www.cancerhelp.org.uk for all the latest news and help in simple, plain English
- only go to experts and demand the best in whatever field you use
- ask for a second opinion
- keep focused on what you are going to do when you recover. Think about your new life, new diet and new sense of purpose
- read this book carefully and keep it to refer to

- Other questions you might want answered are:

- what help and care will Social Services provide?
- am I eligible for any government financial help? Or from any cancer or other charitable organisations?
- how will this affect my private healthcare or my life insurance?
- what difference would it make if I went privately and what would it cost?

- where is the best place and where are the best doctors for my type of cancer?
- is this treatment likely to make me infertile? If so can I do anything about it or about preserving my sperm or eggs?

Doctors have a system for defining how bad the cancer is. You should ask, 'is it a primary and do I have secondaries?'. Cancers are defined in terms of 'grade' and 'stage', each on a 0–4 scale. After a biopsy (or sample) of the tumour is taken, you should be told what 'grade' the cancer is. Low-grade tumours are slower growing and considered less dangerous, but high-grade tumours are deemed aggressive.

The spread of the cancer from its origin is deemed the stage. With a breast cancer for example the spread may be a long way, maybe to the lymph nodes. The maximum grade is 4, meaning widely disseminated. Cancer may spread via the blood or lymph systems.

In the case of many tumours, a lung or whole body X-ray or scan will be taken to see whether the tumour is a primary, or a secondary to a primary in another location.

Finally, blood tests may be used to show evidence of tumours. All this should all be confirmed in a written histology report and you are entitled to a copy. Get hold of this, read it, discuss it with your buddy and your specialist and write an action plan (see next question).

You cannot know too much. Information is power. Remember, in the USA the survival rates are higher than in the UK and one of the major reasons for this, since the treatments themselves are often comparable, is the sheer determination and fighting spirit of the American sufferer. They argue more, demand second opinions, new medicines and drug trials, whatever it takes. The fighting spirit carries them forward and, the fact is, keeps them alive longer. Apparently British sufferers are far too accepting of their fate, 'I have cancer, it's a life-threatening situation but my doctor will do his best for me'.

Do not be like this.

Be determined. Be a fighter and be positive.

187

Q35. How do I improve my chances of being cured?

Up to three quarters of all cancer sufferers in Britain are cured. With some cancers this figure approaches 95 per cent! The definition of a cure used by the medical profession is that the patient did not die from their cancer within five years of being diagnosed.

So, three out of four people with cancer will survive. As I said at the start, the moment you are diagnosed you should immediately start to think:

'How can I improve my odds?'
'How can I move the 75 per cent figure to 100 per cent for me personally?'
Start taking action immediately putting in place the following 'action plan', referring to summary 3 in section V and reading the relevant sections of this book:

- Evaluate your diet, and go on to a strict diet as outlined

- Take a crash course of supplements

- Evaluate your lifestyle
- cut out carcinogens, like drinking, smoking and cosmetics
- take exercise; try yoga and meditation.

- Get support
- contact the cancer helplines
- talk to cranial osteopaths, homeopaths, acupuncturists, visualisers, healers
- have a virus, parasite and yeast check.

- Concentrate on you
- cut all the stresses from your life, be absolutely ruthless about this
- take time for yourself
- find a buddy who will stick with you throughout.

- Be determined
- be absolutely clear. This is a fight to the death. The death of

you or the death of the cancer, and the odds already say you should win. But be determined, be disciplined and really do exactly what is necessary to beat it without cutting corners or making compromises.

- Focus on the future
- when I have beaten this, how is my life going to change? Who do I want to be? What do I want to do? What would I like to have? What would I like to learn?
- give yourself clear and attainable reasons for living and focus on them. Don't just settle for more of the past. Think about your personal development.

Make no mistake, you were no victim unless there was a severe attack of asbestos from your roof, or a leak from the nuclear power station nearby! By and large you contracted cancer because of your own personal habits. Plan ahead, plan to change them to make yourself well, and start now planning the new life you want in five years' time.

The medical profession will now swing into action and it will all happen expertly and very, very quickly. Sometimes it seems, too quickly. Now is the time to plan. Three treatments are the likely options:

- Surgery
- Radiotherapy
- Chemotherapy.

I will deal with each in turn in the following pages.

It may only be days before your surgery. It may be four to 10 weeks before radio or chemotherapy, depending upon the region you are living in and whether you are NHS or private.

Use the time wisely for both short-term and long-term preparation.

Q36. What about a second opinion?

We British hold our doctors in awe. We don't like to upset them so feel that asking for a second opinion is somehow being rude. It isn't.

'I went to my doctor and he said I had cancer; so I asked for a second opinion. OK. You're ugly too.' The comedian Tommy Cooper always had a different way of looking at things. And you must do this too.

Firstly, let me concentrate on the first opinion. Biopsy plus CT or MRI scan and blood tests should give a clear picture of the problem.

- A computed axial tomography (CT or CAT) scan is a 3 D X-ray and takes 20–30 minutes.
- A Magnetic Resonance Imaging (MRI) scan uses a magnetic field instead of X-rays and takes about 30 minutes. Both CTs and MRIs produce a clear and accurate picture of the scene around the tumour and a dye might be injected to show the tumour up more clearly.
- X-rays of other areas of the body may then be taken to discover if there is only one tumour. Armed with all this infor-mation ask the doctor in front of you if they are going to manage your whole recovery process, which may involve surgery, neurology, radiotherapy and chemotherapy. If they are not, then who is?

In the field of cancer, where several treatment options are pos-sible and clearly the patient is in a life threatening situation, it is considered the norm to ask for a second opinion and all the medical records should be made freely available to the patient to pass on to a second expert. It will definitely not be seen as a vote of no confidence, in fact a second opinion is a natural, concerned and intelligent thing to embark on. Your doctor will actually expect you to be interested enough in your own personal welfare to be taking a second opinion, and that second opinion, even if it reaches the same conclusion as the first one, should help you feel more confident about the complete process of treatment.

So how do you find a second opinion?

- You can ask your GP, but they have more than likely referred you to the person they consider to be the best in the first place. You could go to a private GP and ask what they think and for their views on other sources.
- You can search the internet. Many acclaimed international hospitals offer a simple 'send us the information' service.
- Try to get the second opinion from outside of the system that gave you the first. Doctors trained in the same hospital will usually give you the same answers.
- You can telephone a large teaching hospital which will help you establish the top specialists in your type of cancer.
- You can go for a second opinion to the alternative medicine field. If you do, go to someone with a lot of experience in your specific cancer.

Having taken a second opinion discuss it with your original doctor and again prepare an action plan with your buddy.

Q37. Can you tell me about surgery?

Approximately 60 per cent of cancer patients will have surgery. However, it can take several forms.

Some operations may involve **endoscopes** where an instrument is inserted through a hole made in the body. The endoscope allows the surgeon to 'see' inside the body and take a small amount of tissue for examination.

Some operations may involve a similarly small treatment. For example, the majority of bladder cancer only affects the bladder lining and can be removed using a **cytoscope** (a tube passed into the bladder). The bladder can continue to work normally and, even if the cancer returns, it may be possible to work on it again in this way.

Some operations, whilst requiring the surgeon to open up the body, may only be to take tissue for testing. For example, in cases of brain tumours the surgeon may open up the skull, take some tissue from the tumour, and then use titanium screws to hold the skull back in place. At a later date, if there is a need for a full operation, or a second operation, the plate can be lifted.

Surgery in these examples is **diagnostic**. The surgeon uses his skills and, with the aid of the pathology and histology reports, can make an accurate assessment of the problem.

It should be stressed that in the majority of these cases, the results will indicate that the problem is not malignant.

However, after taking samples for test, the tumour may be deemed malignant and the surgeon's role will be crucial in establishing the stage and/or grade of the cancer. Metastasis is the name given to the process by which malignant disease spreads to distant parts of the body, and to the secondary tumours resulting from this process. For example, the rogue cells can circulate in your blood stream to attack cells in your liver or brain, or it is possible that the body's natural defence system will have identified rogue cells and taken them via the lymph to the lymph nodes for examination.

If the tumour is confined to a single site and is whole, like a pea or a ball, it is said to be a **solid tumour**. This is ideal for surgery and the whole tumour may be removed effectively. For example breast, stomach, thyroid, testicular and skin cancers are often tackled in this way. If the primary has been detected early enough, the messages to other parts of the body may be minimal and surgery can be an effective one-stop cure.

If the tumour has started to spread, the surgeon may also remove some of the surrounding tissue. If it has moved to a lymph gland he may well remove that too.

These days, a surgeon would always prefer to confine his surgery to a localised removal e.g. breast lumps or bowel tumours, rather than having to perform radical extensive surgery. The former is clean and limited and considerably improves the quality of the patient's life.

If the cancer has spread, or there is a risk it may have done, surgery may well be followed by radiotherapy and/or chemo-therapy. Further surgery is also a possibility but is only needed in a small number of cases.

There have been debates about whether the action of surgery itself causes the cancer to spread. There was a report in the *Lancet* in 1995 about this possibility with prostate cancer. Anyway the anaesthetic will flatten your immune system and make you more susceptible to the cancer spreading immediately after the surgery, so take positive action to boost your immune system with the ideas in this book.

For a long time there have also been rumblings about the pos-sible dangers of cancer spread when having biopsies (for example, in breast cancer or prostate cancer). The *BMJ* (July 2004) quoted a report from Australian surgeons whose stated view was that 'continuing liver biopsies gave rise to a serious risk of seeding' and was 'useless and dangerous'. No doubt your surgeon will have his own views but be aware that there have been several studies over the years suggesting that fine needles can pick up cancer cells from one location and transport them to another, non-cancerous, one.

Finally remember one important fact. The surgeon will do his level best to cut out all the cancer from your body that he safely can. But it is most likely that your diet, the products you use and your lifestyle brought on the cancer originally. You will ultimately only beat the cancer if you change the habits that gave it to you in the first place. For a short while your life may be in his hands. But in the longer term, it's in your own.

Q38. What should I ask the surgeon?

1. Please describe the operation in detail
2. What are the risks during the operation?
3. What are the risks after the operation?
4. Will surgery cure the problem or merely slow it down?
5. What does the surgeon consider to be success?
6. What are the short-term and long-term side effects?
7. What follow up would be needed after surgery?
8. What if my cancer comes back after surgery?
9. How often has the surgeon performed this particular operation before?
10. What chance is there that the surgery itself may cause the cancer to spread?

The most important thing is to get the best expertise. Common cancers may be treated by oncologists at the patient's local unit. Less common ones should be referred to specialist units and doctors who have a track record in the specific cancer.

It is possible to access the database at the Department of Health or your Local Strategic Health Authority to check out your surgeon. Don't be shy about this, it is your life after all!

Q39. What can I do to recover from surgery quickly?

- Likely scars can be lessened by taking the following supplements daily
  - 2 gms vitamin C (4 x 500 mgs Ester C, time release or at different times of the day)
  - 400 IU vitamin E (you can take up to 1,000 IU)
  - 25 mgs zinc
  - 1,000 mgs of cod liver oil.

- The above supplements may also help your immune system, but you could add the following daily to really boost it:
  - 6 mgs of beta-carotene twice per day
  - 200 mcgs of selenium
  - Drink 6–12 cups of Essiac per day
  - 10–20 mgs of lycopene
  - 30 mgs coenzyme Q10.

There are more suggestions in the answers in Section II.

- The following have an immune boosting effects and specific action on tumours:
  - 2 garlic tablets twice per day
  - 2 gms soya isoflavones per day
  - 2–3 gms astragalus per day.

- Drink 1.5–2.5 litres of good quality water per day to flush the anaesthetic through and take a three to five day detox when you come out of hospital. Buy a simple herbal detox from a pharmacy and read the instructions or ask the pharmacist.

- Toxins can be removed from the alimentary canal by adding 2 tablespoons of linusit (organic linseeds) to your breakfast cereal and taking 1,500 mgs of psyllium seeds each day. If you increase your fibre intake you should increase your zinc intake to 50 mgs as fibre prevents zinc absorption, and you must drink lots of water with both.

- If the tumour was in the brain take 500–1,500 mgs of soya

lecithin per day as this contains choline and inositol, two B vitamins which cross the blood/brain barrier and nourish brain cells. Soya lecithin will help all your cell membranes, and your liver.

- Take a multivitamin and multimineral complex preferably in colloidal form and containing iron to help in blood regeneration. The B vitamins it contains will also help to overcome the stress of the operation and aid the healing process, for example, biotin will help the action of vitamin C and folic acid will help your DNA replicate correctly.

After the operation, massage the scar gently with vitamin E cream. Arnica is also supposed to help.

Manual lymphatic drainage (MLD)

- Lymphoedema is a chronic swelling due to a failure of lymph drainage. It can sometimes occur after cancer surgery where the adjacent lymph nodes have been removed or radiated. If the lymph nodes under the arm have been surgically removed following breast cancer, this can result in a swollen arm. After testicular or prostate cancer treatment, removal of the nodes in the groin can cause swollen legs or abdomen.
- Lymphoedema is not curable, and if left untreated can lead to many problems including an increase in the size of the limb, or torso, and a hardening of the tissues (fibrosis), which can impede most of the lymph flow. The area becomes vulnerable to infection and can result in a painful inflammatory condition called cellulites.
- Manual lymphatic drainage (MLD) is an acknowledged therapy for helping to control and maintain lymphoedema, and is used together with skin care, exercises and breathing techniques. The therapist uses very gentle, precise hand movements to accelerate the flow of lymph through the lymphatic system. This results in a softening of the tissues, reduced swelling and a reduction in pain. When the normal drainage route has been destroyed by surgery or radiation it is possible to pump the lymphatic fluid towards functioning lymph vessels for them to take up the extra load, leading to a reduction of

196

the swelling. The gentle pumping action of MLD is used to great advantage to reduce the appearance of scars.

- When necessary, MLD is combined with compression bandaging and exercises designed to prevent the fluid returning to the area. After several treatments, dramatic improvements in swelling are often achieved. When the swelling has reduced, a maintenance programme of treatments is begun and the therapist can supply compression stockings or sleeves if needed. MLD is a deeply relaxing and soothing treatment.
- MLD therapists will give advice on treatment plans, skin care, exercises and self-massage where appropriate, and will liaise with the patient's doctor/consultant to ensure the best possible outcome. In the UK, there are several recognized training schools for MLD including Vodder, Asdonk, Le Duc, Foldi and Casely-Smith and it is vital that the therapist is properly trained.

Herbs and supplements

Some herbal remedies such as garlic, ginseng and ginkgo may interfere with clotting mechanisms. The problem is that: *"There is no reliable guidance for surgeons and anaesthetists. The research is incomplete,"* says Professor Edzard Ernst Director of Complementary Medicine at Exeter University. 'What about patients?' I am inclined to ask!

Calendula taken a week before through to a week after surgery can reduce the side effects of anaesthetic, limit inflammation and reduce scarring. Arnica can be taken immediately after surgery to improve healing and reduce bruising and blood loss; staphysagria, a few days later if the wound is particularly bad.

Q40. Can you tell me about radiotherapy?

In an earlier answer the effect of free radicals damaging DNA was covered. If the configuration of the DNA is changed it is extremely likely that a nonsensical code sequence will be produced and the body's natural defence system will throw it out. Radiotherapy adopts the same principle, attempting to similarly change the DNA, albeit this time in a rogue cell, so that it becomes gobbledegook, is neutralised and similarly taken away by the body's natural defences.

Radiotherapy uses high speed ionising radiation similar to X-rays to hit the DNA in abnormal cells. To have an effect it must hit the DNA when it is dividing. Radiotherapy is very successful at screwing up this division, causing the copy to be full of errors. The radiation uses lasers fired from very large, very sophisticated machines and can be targeted very accurately.

The effectiveness of radiotherapy has to be balanced by the risks but, essentially, depending upon the grade, stage and type of cancer, radiotherapy can be very effective. But please note that the activity of the radiotherapy continues for up to four to six weeks after the radiation sessions have finished..

A little more detail

The higher the energy of the ionising rays, the deeper into the body the rays can go.

A package of energy is a 'photon' and this is divided into 'fractions'. Whilst X-rays were the first type used, these are now often replaced by gamma rays. Particle beam radiation using fast moving subatomic particles can also be used to treat localised cancers.

Internal radiotherapy involves placing small radioactive pellets or implants into the localised tumour to do the damage.

Techniques are being developed all the time in an attempt to kill more of the cancers' cells and less of the surrounding good guys. Radiosensitisers make the tumour more susceptible to damage from radiotherapy; radioprotectors protect the normal cells. Radio labelled antibodies are also being used as cancer seekers.

Radiotherapy is a very targeted and localised treatment. When treatment is considered, a patient will firstly go through a planning stage, lying under a simulator which takes X-rays of the area to be treated. In this way the medical team can target the tumour accurately and plan how to stay focused on that area, whilst moving the angle of attack to minimise damage to a healthy area adjacent to the tumour. Each session of radiotherapy is very short, just a few minutes, although radiotherapy may be required over a number of weeks. Radiotherapy is not painful.

The total dosage is very carefully calculated to do the most efficient and effective job so the patient must go to every planned session and avoid missing any. Apparently (and somewhat nonsensically) only about 20 per cent of patients go to all the treatments. One reason is the patient's depression, which is quite normal and can set in after a couple of weeks.

Sometimes one big dose is given rather than small does (stereotactic radiotherapy), depending upon the type of cancer and how far it has spread.

Radiotherapy is becoming more and more sophisticated, and is the medical profession's front line weapon in treating cancers effectively. In some cancer tumours, it definitely does work but, because of the free radical action on the surrounding tissues, there is a small chance of contracting a second completely new cancer from the radiation itself. Ask about this.

Q41. What side-effects are there to radiotherapy?

These depend upon the exact type of cancer and the location.

- If the rogue cells are not dividing – and at any one time they will not all be doing so – they won't be affected. This is the 'Achilles heel' of radiotherapy.
- Other nearby healthy cells that are dividing can be damaged or killed. Often the healthy cells that are damaged belong to the blood supply system or membrane structure. The theory is that these normal cells will be regenerated in time, but this is not always the case. In the case of breast cancer, sometimes up to 15 per cent of lung tissue is permanently damaged in this way.
- The area may get a little 'burned', so bright sunshine on the skin should be avoided. The area attacked should be washed only in cold water and aloe vera gel used.
- Hair loss may well occur in the direct line of the beam but the hair will return.
- Radiation weakens the body overall. Both the blood and lymph cells are attacked by radiotherapy, reducing the numbers of both red and white blood cells. The liver also works overtime removing dead cells and toxins.
- Most patients get very tired and should plan to sleep or simply rest for a couple of hours per day. Fatigue can be a real problem and Italian doctors have identified the cause as low levels of carnitine circulating in the blood stream. They recommend taking energy drinks with supplements of carnitine. Apparently in research energy levels came back within one week for 90 per cent of patients. The tiredness will probably extend to lethargy and patients may also feel sick. Travelling long distances to the hospital may be tiring and the location of the treatment centre and its distance from where you stay the night need to be given some thought.
- Drinking peppermint tea may calm the stomach and help the nausea that affects some people.

The number of blood cells is called your blood count and this should be monitored carefully throughout radiotherapy. Radio-therapy must be stopped if the blood count falls too far.

- In extreme cases, radiotherapy can lead to sterility.
- Some people may suffer from mouth ulcers. If so, avoid all sugar and salt, calm your stomach with peppermint tea and avoid stress and acid foods.
- After about two weeks of treatment and again about two weeks after finishing treatment, the patient may suffer acute depression and it is at this point the buddy and family members, friends and partners need to rally round. Don't be embarrassed to ask someone to watch over you during this time. Going alone to radiotherapy in week three when you are tired and depressed can be a very lonely experience, so take someone with you. But you must keep up treatments and avoid missing any sessions.
- There is some evidence that radiotherapy, whilst it cures the first cancer, can cause long term problems in the surrounding healthy cells. Patients treated for cervical cancer can show major urinary problems 25 years later. Lung tissues are especially susceptible to radiation damage. In one research report, 19 of 31 breast cancer patients went on to get lung cancer, on average 17 years later.

Q42. What should I ask the doctor in charge?

1. What would the doctor consider to be a successful response at the end of the radiotherapy treatment?

   – no cancer tumour remaining?
   – tumour present but much smaller?
   – other?

2. How long will the treatment be? Will you be an outpatient or inpatient? Is this a one-off treatment, or might there be more?

3. What is the doctor's success rate, and how does that compare to the national average?

4. How often has the doctor personally treated your type of tumour?

5. What do they consider the next step after radiotherapy, and why?

6. What happens if there is no response? How often does that occur? What is the fallback plan?

7. What exactly do they think the side effects are likely to be?

8. What are the chances of each side effect?

9. What supplements would they recommend to improve

   – the success of the radiotherapy?
   – the reduction of side effects?
   – the speed of recovery?

Q43. How can I protect myself from the side-effects of radiotherapy?

We have already covered the fact that radiotherapy is going to attack all rapidly dividing cells in the line of fire. So it will attack the rapidly dividing cells adjacent to the cancer, flatten your blood count and lymph systems, and thus your immune system. It will fill the body, and especially the liver, with toxins and dead cells.

This means you have to have an action plan to try to keep yourself as strong as possible throughout. A major problem here is that some of the vitamins and supplements you might still wish to take to maintain your immune system will also inhibit the action of the radiotherapy by protecting the very cells it should be attacking.

Everything you can take is explained more fully in section II. So this section is intended to be little more than a checklist. From the start you should consider yoga and meditation, and using cranial osteopaths, acupuncturists and healers, to strengthen the immune system and aid your mind-energy-healing link.

It should be stressed up front, that three supplements in particular seem to have a proven record in making radiotherapy more effective. these are:

- Selenium
- Isoflavones (soya or citrus)
- Astragalus.

Some cancer clinics recommend taking vitamin D as well. The suggested action plan divides into three stages and focuses on supplements as a way of kick-starting the health boosting plan. You may prefer to take less supplements and strengthen your diet in the ways I have previously outlined. A full diet is in section V.

(i) Pre-radiotherapy

As soon as you find out you have cancer you should:

- Go to a cranial osteopath and/or acupuncturist to balance and strengthen your body energy systems
- Start a yoga course and, if you feel up to it, maintain a light exercise programme. Learn to meditate.

- Take a multivitamin and mineral complex, ideally in a colloidal form, which includes some iron and B complex with at least 400 mcgs of folic acid
- Take

Beta-carotene	6 mgs twice per day
Vitamin C	500 mgs four times per day
Vitamin E	400 IU daily
Zinc	25 mgs daily
Selenium	200 mcgs daily
Coenzyme Q10	30 mgs daily
Lycopene	10–20 mgs daily

all of which will strengthen your immune system.

- Take 1,000 mgs of fish oil and 2 garlic tablets daily or eat lots of oily fish and raw garlic. Take 3,000 mgs astragalus and drink Essiac tea. Replace all drinks of tea, coffee and chocolate with green tea.
- Take an amino acid supplement containing glutamine. This stimulates the liver to produce glutathione, which is very strong in repairing damaged cells, and L-cysteine, which is particularly important in DNA repair. Alternatively, instead of taking the supplements, eat the foods in which they are naturally found. Glutathione is present in fruit and vegetables especially raw carrots, asparagus, avocado and cruciferous vegetables (e.g. Brussel sprouts, cabbage, broccoli). Glutathione levels may be enhanced by taking polysaccharides like Aloe Vera, or Ambrotose. L-cysteine is found in kelp (seaweed), eggs and garlic.
- Switch away from all dairy products and consider using GM-free soya milk. Take 3 gms per day of soya lecithin, which has an excellent content of inositol and choline, as it is a fat emulsifier and will help the liver break down the excess fats lying there. Add to this 2 gms per day of soya isoflavones. This will help in all cases of hormone induced cancer.
- Detox. Buy a proprietary detox from a health store and use it for at least four days to help clean the liver.
- Drink 1.5–3 litres of pure water, which will also help clear away the toxins and clean the liver.

- Take 200 mgs per day of milk-thistle to strengthen your liver.
- Always avoid animal fats, saturated oils and dairy products as cancer cells thrive on fats.

(ii) During radiotherapy and for four to six weeks after

- Keep the momentum of the pre-radiotherapy stage going
- in terms of visits to the cranial osteopath/acupuncturist, regular yoga and meditation. But you will probably be too tired for regular light exercise;
- take all the supplements including the antioxidants beta-carotene, vitamin C, lycopene, Essiac and coenzyme Q10;
- ensure you do take the selenium, soya isoflavones and astragalus as all three have been proven to make radiotherapy work more effectively;
- detox after three weeks, six weeks and nine weeks if you feel up to it;
- continue drinking 1.5–3 litres of water and avoiding fats and oils;
- Take carnitine.

This stage should continue for at least four to six weeks after the radiotherapy finishes as the action of the radiotherapy is still taking place although treatments have stopped. If you haven't felt up to it before, you should try to do a proper detox prior to starting Stage (iii).

(iii) Post-radiotherapy

- Keep all of the above going.
- Take a supplement of organic iron for just one week at the start to raise your blood count.
- Take 1,500 mgs of echinacea and 1,000 mgs of cat's claw (Uno de Gato), the latter taken on an empty stomach, along with the 3,000 mgs of astragalus, all of which help to regenerate a healthy immune system quickly. See answer 19 for more details on herbal immune boosters.

Yes, you are taking a lot of pills, which you should spread out during the day. You can of course eat the natural alternative to some of the above and prepare wonderful fresh juices, but the supplement volumes above are 'insurance' amounts designed to give you the best possible chance of beating the cancer. A summary diet plan is contained in section VI.

Remember the latest research evidence from the USA, and experts such as Boik at MD Anderson is that supplementation (use natural products where possible) actually helps the success of radiotherapy. And in this book, we like 'help'!

Q44. Can you tell me about chemotherapy?

Chemotherapy, historically, has involved the use of chemicals to poison rogue cells, typically rapidly dividing cells, usually poisoning them through free radical toxic action.

The drugs used will vary according to the type of tumour and its state of advancement. Some chemicals work directly on the cell. Some work on the receptors at the cell surface and try to stop the rogue messages taking hold.

The risks are in the side effects. Chemotherapy historically has been a very general treatment. Too general. Rather like trying to kill a terrorist gang in a city with an air borne bombing raid. You may kill them, some may escape, but some innocent bystanders may suffer too.

Pills taken orally or drugs administered into veins poison the whole body. The liver and immune system do their best to remove the poisons, but both are weakened severely in the process. Other rapidly dividing cells, such as those in the nails, blood, stomach lining and hair, also suffer. Often sickness is a real problem, as it further debilitates the patient. During the chemotherapy the blood count declines and less oxygen is carried round the body. Often after a couple of weeks, and again around week six, the patient gets depressed. One reason is that the blood oxygen level and depression are directly linked. It can happen in reverse; depressed people have lower levels of oxygen carried in their blood streams.

Estimates suggest that, on average, 10 per cent of patients who have undergone typical chemotherapy ultimately contract a completely new unrelated cancer at a later date, caused by the chemotherapy toxins damaging DNA in other cells. This estimate appears low according to recent research. Studies now show, for example, that one third of female childhood cancer survivors suffer a breast cancer by the time they are 40 years old. Indeed, amongst women in their late 20s and 30s, breast cancer is 16 times more common than the norm where chemotherapy was administered to them as children. Nearly one quarter of patients treated with anthracyclines go on to develop heart problems, with women being particularly affected.

Chemotherapy success rates vary dramatically. In child leukaemias chemotherapy has a good record, as it does, for example, with testicular cancer. But for brain tumours, *The Lancet* in February 2004 reported that drugs do not work at all.

A survey of 128 US cancer doctors found that if they themselves contracted cancer over 80 per cent would not resort to chemotherapy as the 'risks and side effects far outweighed the likely benefits'. What they would actually do if they had cancer is possibly another matter.

In a little more detail

Barely a week seems to go by without a new magic drug going through trials. No wonder in the USA alone the industry is a $7bn business.

There are a lot of drugs, all different and for different situations. Increasingly scientists are trying to localise the drug to the tumour. This is because when a pill is taken orally, or a drug intravenously, it spreads right round the body. The liver, for example, tries to expel it and so only a small percentage actually reaches the target; resulting in high wastage of the drug and random damage to the patient's body. This explains why the recipient can feel so ill, tired, depressed and why the liver and kidneys become so poisoned.

To illustrate current thinking and progress being made, here are some examples:

- Temozolomide is a new drug just given FDA approval to treat astrocytomas (Grade 3 brain tumours). It has been used on patients where the tumours have reappeared after radiotherapy and chemotherapy have failed. In tests amongst 54 patients, seven had tumours that shrunk and five had their tumours disappear. So a 9 per cent success rate and a 22 per cent effect. Possible side effects are headaches, nausea, fatigue and low blood counts. However the 'clinical trials' provided no information on the drug's long-term success or safety
- Thalidomide is making a serious comeback. Already approved

in certain countries for use with multiple myeloma, Cancer Research UK is now investigating its benefits with certain lung cancers. One of its 'benefits' is that it can stop blood vessel growth. Pregnant women will not be allowed in the trial.

- The FDA has approved a 'wafer impregnated with a drug that is inserted next to the actual brain tumour'. This treatment, which fights Grade 4 glioblastoma multiforme and is called Gliadel, delivers the anti-cancer drug Carmustine directly to the tumour site in higher concentration. The six-month survival rate amongst 222 adults went up from 36 per cent with placebo to 56 per cent with Gliadel.

- There are trials being conducted in America using Toxin Therapy, for example, where a poisonous bacterium (in this case *Pseudomanas bacteriae*) is armed with an anti-cancer drug (Interleukin 4) and only attacks and kills cancer cells but not the patient's healthy ones.

- Gleevec is a drug recently developed, which blocks a cellular receptor enzyme. When a rogue messenger hits a cell it has to be shunted through 58 receptors until it reaches the nucleus and can cause its havoc. Gleevec was developed to block that process. Although the drug was developed for use with brain tumours (it was originally called Glivac), it doesn't seem to work with them. However it was found to work with chronic myeloid leukaemia and the FDA has given its approval for the use of the drug with this disease.

By now you should be getting the picture. Vast effort, lots of different drugs, formats and applications. Low returns but increasing sophistication.

Chemotherapy is also increasingly used to reduce the size of tumours thus enabling surgery or radiotherapy which previously might have been impossible. This clearly has significant benefits. Against these must be weighed a report (*Journal of Nat. Cancer Inst.* 2005; 97) from the Ionnina School of Medicine in Greece where a study of 9 previous studies incorporating 4000 breast cancer patients concluded that such use of 'prior chemo' to shrink tumours resulted in 22 per cent more tumours after treatment!

Guided Missiles

If the American Army scientists can pick off one house in a whole city with a smart bomb, the challenge is there for the medical scientists too. And they are responding, albeit slowly. For example:

- A whole new breed of drugs for breast cancer sufferers looks to cut the driving force behind the disesase; namely too much oestrogen. Drugs called aromatase inhibitors seek to reduce oestogen levels in females. A similar pattern is emerging with males and prostate cancer. There, Finasteride and ICI and just two drugs to cut oestrogen levels in men now that the hormone has been found guilty of driving prostate cancer.
- Scientists are also developing ways of helping the immune system better detect and neutralise rogue cells. In the Patterson Institute in Manchester, scientists have been taking blood from bowel cancer patients, removing the T-cells, engineering them with an artificial gene which directs them at the cancer, then putting the modified T-cells back into the patient. Apparently it works 100 per cent of the time in the laboratory.
- Finally scientists are also homing in on what differentiates a cancer cell from a normal cell; like the unique enzymes in the power stations, or genetic differences. In a healthy cell the p53 gene protects the cell's DNA, but in a cancer cell it is turned off, while other genes cause the cancer cell to grow and divide uncontrollably. Scientists are exploring ways of reversing this and re-energising the p53 protective gene.

All in all be absolutely sure you know what your chemotherapy drug is supposed to do, and how it is going to do it.

Do not rush in to chemotherapy without knowing all the facts. If your doctor recommends chemotherapy make sure you know everything about the drug he is suggesting. You will find new drugs covered on the internet complete with results of their trials. Or you can ask a professional complementary centre like the Bristol Cancer Help Centre or your specific cancer charity/foundation helpline and also get a second opinion. (The very latest cancer treatments can be obtained on the Medcast Web site – http:// webmd-practice.medcast.com/smed/web).

You may like to re-read the short pieces of information on both carctol and MGN-3 with a view to taking either during chemotherapy. Carctol is probably more of an all-round alkaliser, while MGN-3 is more specific to boosting the immune system even during chemotherapy, whilst reducing side effects. Also vitamins K1 and K2 have been listed to improve chemotherapy effectiveness (Yoshida et al, Tokyo Medical University), and we now know that antioxidants and many vitamins and minerals can actually help the success rate of chemotherapy, as is covered elsewhere in this book. Diet is crucial. But, as we found in a report on chemotherapy and diet for **icon**, diets in hospitals are prepared by dieticians and targeted at patients facing extreme weight loss. This accounts for about ten per cent of all cases. Visit our website for more explanation and to review the arguments against the often recommended high sugar, high dairy, high fat and calorie hospital recommendations. Also look for information on 'Hydrazine Sulphate' which in Russian clinical trials, not only combats weight loss, but aids chemotherapy and improves 'cure' rates.

Finally, two words of warning. Firstly a lady with breast cancer who was talking to us told us how horrified she was to discover that various of her drugs (for sleeping and nausea) contained lactose, when she had deliberately tried to have a dairy free diet. Read all labels carefully.

Secondly, some complementary treatments, particularly extracts and herbs, may affect the action of prescribed chemotherapy drugs. You should tell your specialist exactly what else you are doing for treatment and seek advice on possible reactions between the treatments. If he criticises a herb or complementary therapy, please ask to see the evidence. Subjectivity is the enemy of success.

Q45. What questions should I ask my doctor about chemotherapy?

1. How long has the doctor been prescribing this course of treatment, and how many people have undergone the treatment?
2. Exactly how does this drug work?
3. If they had your cancer, would they treat themselves with this drug?
4. How many cases have they treated with this drug, and what has the success rate been? (Define success!)
5. What are the alternatives?
6. What is the fall back if it doesn't work?
7. Does the doctor expect the tumour to go, or just to reduce in size? What are the chances of either happening?
8. What are the risks in having the treatment?
9. What are the short and long-term side effects during and after the treatment?
10. What diet and other alternative therapies does your doctor recommend to help minimise the side effects?

Q46. How do I best recover from chemotherapy?

As we have seen, most chemotherapy works rather like radio-therapy in that it tries to kill off rapidly dividing cancer cells by poisoning them with an excess of free radicals. Unfortunately these free radicals can cause you a lot of damage. The problem with trying to define a recovery programme is that specific drugs might cause specific problems or require specific solutions to return your system back to health. Most of the general recommendations to answer this question are common to Q 41.

Whilst the chemotherapy is going on you should drink up to 3 litres of water, eat as nourishingly as you can, avoiding fats where possible, (a carbohydrate based diet is best), and consider taking 400 IU vitamin E, 200 mcgs selenium, 3000 mgs of astragalus and 2 gms soya isoflavones to help the effectiveness of the treatment. You should avoid all alcohol as your liver certainly needs no more toxins at the moment, and take milk thistle (*Silybum marianum*) (200 mgs) and soya lecithin to help to 'de-fat' it and strengthen it.

When the chemotherapy has finished, its action may well continue for weeks, and you should ask your doctor about this. There are so many different chemotherapy drugs it is impossible to generalise.

However, you need to rebuild your immune and energy systems as fast as possible. For example:

- Get a cranial osteopath to rebalance your energy and think about going to see an acupuncturist. Take a simple detox for about three days to try and clean up your system and ease back into vitamin C (4 x 500 gms) and beta-carotene (2 x 6 mgs) plus CoQ10 (30 mgs).
- Throughout the whole chemotherapy period take zinc (25 mgs) and cod liver oil (1,000 mgs) and a colloidal multivitamin and mineral supplement with good levels of vitamin B and folic acid. If the multivitamin contained iron it might be a benefit. Firstly, iron actually seems to enhance the activity of the free

radicals and so it might help the chemotherapy. Secondly, it will help boost the blood count, which has taken a hammering.

- Astragalus, cat's claw, echinacea and Essiac are all mentioned elsewhere and may be taken after chemotherapy to re-stimulate the immune system.
- People over 35 may take wild yam to boost their DHEA levels, and eat salads and carbohydrate in the evening (carbohydrates and salads aid seratonin production, which in turn stimulates melatonin levels). Older people might even think about taking a small dose of melatonin supplement if their doctor agrees, or ornithine and argenine to stimulate Hgh.
- As with radiotherapy, you must also stimulate your body and mind.

Remember. It is a proven fact that visualisation, yoga and meditation all help boost the immune system and have a significant effect on long-term survival rates.

Fatigue

Fatigue comes free with every chemotherapy treatment. The usual recommendation is to surrender and rest.

However, research by Italian scientists (Graziano, Milan 2002), has identified that it is linked to loss of carnitine in the blood, as a result of the chemotherapy toxins.

In tests, albeit involving just 50 patients given a high energy drink contain levocarnitine (which is converted to carnitine in the body), 45 of the patients no longer felt fatigue within just one week of starting the drink. Talk to your doctor about this research.

Anaemia

Two recent studies presented at the European Society for Medical Oncology (October 2004) concluded that epoetins had a major benefit for people suffering from anaemia during chemotherapy. The first study showed that with solid tumours the risk of death was reduced by 51 per cent in those patients whose anaemia was managed by epoetins. The second study showed that epoetins reduced the risk of tumour progression.

SECTION V

Specific cancers and
the coming cancer cures

Introduction

We will now look at some of the leading cancers and what research shows might help, whilst hopefully maintaining the 'easy to read' tone of this book. More information will be found on our website www.iconmag.co.uk.

Q47. Can you tell me a few things specific to my cancer?

It is not the purpose of this book to provide detailed views of every cancer. More, this book is about general principles. However, below we will cover some of the main cancers and pass on some of the latest research information; much of which your doctor may not yet know. Yet more information is available, free, on www.iconmag.co.uk. I suggest you read all of the following, even if you do not have that particular cancer, as many helpful hints cross to other cancers

• Prostate cancer

Many men are told by their doctor that high testosterone levels cause their prostate cancer. Yet in November 2003, the leading UK charity was simply stating 'We do not know the cause'.

Neither of these is true.

For 15 years or more we have known that certain toxic chemicals mimic the action of oestrogen in the body, and that these oestrogen mimics have been very damaging to male genitalia, for example reducing sperm counts by 50 per cent over the last 50 years.

The NCI and the Cancer Prevention Coalition in the USA have done a lot of work on this, as has the Athlone Institute of Technology in Ireland.

In 2002 and 2003 reports from the Singapore National Cancer Centre, the Monash Cancer Institute and the Concord Centre in Sydney, Australia, all reported that localised oestrogen was causal to prostate cancer. Research also showed that both testosterone and oestrogen were 'needed' for prostate cancer.

Dr Thomson of the Texas Cancer Centre in Houston solved the riddle when he proved that testosterone did not cause cancer (and anyway there has never been a study where testosterone added to cells in vitro caused cancer, unlike oestrogen). He showed that oestrogen could turn 'safe' testosterone into DHT, which is an extremely aggressive agent.

Since testosterone declines with age, it was unlikely to be causal anyway.

Men do make more oestrogen nowadays largely through poor eating habits (for example, high animal fat content leads to more steroid production) and through simply being overweight. A fat post-menopausal woman can have more oestrogen in her body than a thin pre-menopausal one; a fat 55-year-old male, more than his 40-year-old wife. Males can also ingest more of it through the animal fat they eat or via recycled tap water in cities (thanks to all those ladies on HRT and the pill!). But another boost to their 'oestrogen pool' has been through their use of toxic toiletries, household products and their ingestion of pesticides and herbicides. Many of these mimic oestrogen once in the bloodstream.

Far more on this subject can be found in my book, *Oestrogen: The Killer in Our Midst*.

In a recorded conversation I asked the helpline of a key charity how to prevent prostate cancer, given that 'my father and brother had had it and I was over 50' (This was invented but would have made me high risk.)

Their answer was that I should eat more tomatoes and dietary fibre and less animal fat. And go for regular digital rectal examinations. I could have an annual PSA test.

They could have told me the following:

The key problem in the Western world is that every man over 50 seems to have an enlarged prostate. This is mainly due to our diet, an excess of animal fats and particularly dairy, shown in research to promote prostate cell proliferation. The symptoms of an enlarged prostate and prostate cancer are extremely similar (frequency of urination, unempty bladder, etc).

A digital rectal examination will only tell you that you have an enlarged prostate. You will be sent for a PSA test if enlargement is found. A high PSA reading indicates cancer, but drinking milk or taking exercise, for example, before the test can artificially increase the reading. The Fred Hutchinson Cancer Research Centre in Seattle have estimated that PSA screening may over-diagnose prostate cancer by 40 per cent. Sloan-Kettering in New York showed that a one-off PSA test was 'almost useless'. Even scans may be sightly misleading.

A biopsy may be taken but this is a very serious operation and may itself result in impotency and infection.

Worse still, it is becoming clear that many men may be putting themselves at unnecessary risk of serious side effects (e.g. impotence and incontinence) by opting for radical surgery. An American charity has stated that as many as two thirds of prostate operations are probably unnecessary. The Royal Marsden confirms that as many as half of all men diagnosed should not have surgery but instead undergo a programme of 'active surveillance'.

The hardest challenge for doctors is to decide whether the prostate cancer is slow growing or fast growing. In some cases even very small cancers can be fast growing and a new test for this is being developed in the UK, measuring proteins from cancer cells. As yet trials are imperfect.

Given the serious possible side effects from both operations and chemical treatments, prostate treatment should never be rushed into. This is the advice of both UK and US charities. Some things you can do are:

a) Eat tomatoes (lycopene). Harvard Medical School have concluded that 7–10 helpings (especially cooked) per week reduces risk by 40 per cent, and reduces symptoms by the same amount. Lycopene binds to and neutralises circulating "bad" fats in blood.

b) Take saw palmetto oil. Studies show this reduces the size of an enlarged prostate.

c) Take wild yam, a natural source of progesterone which can displace and reduce levels of oestrogen in the body.

d) Lose weight; overweight men have higher oestrogen levels.

e) Reduce consumption of red meats and all animal fats as these will increase oestrogen levels.

f) Take selenium; associated with a 40 per cent lowered risk of cancer.

g) Eat more broccoli. I3C converts the dangerous form of oestrogen (oestradiol) into a safer version (oestrone).

h) Cut out dairy; Swedish studies show a direct correlation between increased risk of prostate and the volume of dairy consumed.

i) Increase intake of vitamin D (sunshine on the body makes

vitamin D from cholesterol – the pigmentation of black people prevents this and may be a reason why black people have higher prostate risk). Fish oils are a good source (but not cod liver oil).

j) Use glass bottled water or install a reverse osmosis water filter if you live in a city.

k) Fred Hutchinson Cancer Centre have also shown a definitive link between high calorie intake and prostate cancer.

l) The good news according to researchers in Boston (*Journal of American Medical Association*) is that regular sex seems to help protect men from prostate cancer.

The Mayo Clinic in 2000 and the original work on eicosanoids by Sir John Vane (1977–82) shows that both taking omega 3 and aspirin (81 mgs only) daily can reduce risk by 40 per cent.

Experts at the University of Pittsburg have shown that men with prostate cancer are twice as likely to carry the cold sore herpes virus. Risk is greater amongst smokers who have increased rates of vitually all cancers.

New drugs like ICI and Finnasteride have shown an ability to reduce prostate size by cutting oestrogen levels in men. Recent research from the University of Illinois (June 2004) shows that simultaneously consuming broccoli plus tomatoes can be more effective than taking Finnasteride at reducing and slowing the growth of tumours.

Clean up your bathroom and your kitchen too – go toxin and oestrogen-mimic free.

A new trial in the UK is about to take place. This trial uses sound waves, which apparently heat the tumour rapidly to 90°C and melt it away! Research has already taken place in Japan with a 70 per cent all clear after five years and only 22 per cent of men complaining of sexual dysfunction (**icon** – 2005 Issue 1). These figures are considerably better than those of current conventional therapies.

• **Breast cancer**

The great majority of breast cancers are hormonally driven by the 'oestrogen pool'. A few are not hormonally driven and are usually caused by extreme toxic poisoning. (A very few breast cancers are linked to the herpes virus after exposure to chicken pox or shingles). Recent research (**icon** – August 2003) showed that women with breast cancer have higher pesticide residues in their bloodstream, a second study showed they had low levels of vitamin B-12, a third that they had low omega 3 levels and a fourth that they had low vitamin C levels.

But breast cancer is most usually due to one main factor. Excess oestrogen. It increases the density of breast tissue and dense breast tissue is risky breast tissue.

One in eight women in the Western world will get breast cancer. This figure increases by 26 per cent for women who take HRT, or have ever taken the pill.

Overweight women seriously increase their risk of breast cancer as do women that over-eat. Animal fats and carbo-hydrates, in excess, both stimulate oestrogen production as does regular alcohol consumption.

Salt and sugar consumption can increase oestrogen levels through their influence on other hormone levels such as insulin.

Dairy consumption is a negative influence whilst soy, or soya, consumption is a positive influence. The 2002 research study in Singapore by three top cancer bodies seals this view. Phytoestro-gens from soy, red clover and pulses like chickpeas, although weaker in their effect than human oestrogen, are sufficiently simi-lar in biochemical structure to be able to bind to receptor sites on healthy cells whilst having no carcinogenic effect. This action blocks the receptors from accepting oestradiol, which can stimu-late breast cancer.

A bigger picture has to be looked at when considering breast cancer.

Centuries ago women had less periods, because of lifestyle and dietary factors. Periods occurred between the ages of 18–38, and more babies and breast feeding periods of up to two years cut the number of monthly oestrogen bursts from today's levels of around 440 per lifetime to around 240.

Higher consumption of animal fats and alcohol, aided and abetted by smoking, worsens this. Significantly lower levels of vegetable, fruit, and pulse consumption provides less protection, whilst high levels of dairy consumption in the West are clearly implicated. (Pulses including soy are known to lengthen the monthly cycle and reduce the total oestrogen levels.)

But the problems do not stop there for women.

Recycled water in cities contains oestrogen residues, and they are constantly exposed to oestrogen mimics in the environment, for example, volatile organic carbon compounds leaching from carpets to computers, from cleaning agents to furniture polish, from breathing petrol fumes to certain perfumes on the skin.

Neither self-examination nor mammograms have been conclusively shown to reduce death rates from the disease; in fact it is arguable that mammograms can actually worsen the overall risk of breast cancer. Research in the USA in 2002 cast serious doubt on even the validity of their results. The European Conference in 2004 concluded they were only 59 per cent accurate for the majority of women, who have dense breast tissue.

As stated earlier in this book, there is also serious concern that half of the 'cancers' diagnosed by mammograms are not cancers at all but DCIS calciferous deposits. A UCLA research study concluded that only 20 per cent of these at most became a cancer. Yet on my speaking tour of the UK, some women in the audience had already been given radiotherapy, whilst others had been diagnosed correctly. Be sure you do have a cancer and do not be rushed.

However it must be noted that early diagnosis is vital. UK research (Coleman, LSHTM) has suggested that higher 5-year survival in the USA (89 per cent against 79 per cent across Europe and 73 per cent in the UK) may be linked to early stage levels of 41 per cent in the USA compared with just 29 per cent in Europe.

Thermal imaging (**icon** – 2005 Issue 1) is a non-invasive and highly accurate diagnostic system. It seems to completely outperform mammograms in accuracy and without safety doubts. Unfortunately there are only four centres in the UK using it.

What is a girl to do?

a) Well if you don't want more children, you could certainly breast feed your babies longer. Not least of all because breast fed children have less illness and higher IQs!

b) Cut dairy, ideally completely.
c) Cut animal fats and excess refined carbohydrates.
d) Do not be overweight.
e) Do not smoke, never take the pill or HRT.
f) Try natural progesterone creams and supplements.
g) Use glass bottled water, or a reverse osmosis filter for all water supplies (including cooking and hot drinks).
h) Eat more fresh vegetables and fruit. More pulses. Women with the highest consumption of soya have less breast cancer (Cancer Research UK/Sloan-Kettering).
i) Eat more garlic – found in the Iowa study to reduce cancer in women.
j) Take tocotrienol vitamin E as it has been shown to out-perform even tamoxifen. The USA is the best source for such supplements as tocopherol vitamin E dominates Europe and this is not so effective. Tocotrienols are found in palm oil and collect in breast tissue, reducing density.
k) Vitamin B-12 deficiency appears linked to folic acid deficiency and women with breast cancer have lower B-12 levels. Supplement (chlorella is a good source of B-12).
l) In fact women with the highest levels of omega 3 in their circulation have no breast cancer. Good vitamin A levels are also important.
m) Eat organic and fresh. Pesticides and some preservatives, like parabens in toiletries and suncreams, increase oestrogen levels and have been found in malignant breast tissue.
n) Clean out the toxic products and oestrogen mimic chemicals from your bathroom, your make-up and your kitchen.

Some women will be identified as higher risk; women who have a mother or sister with the disease. They can also be identified with certain genes.

BRCA1 damage allows cancer cells to hide from immune system searching cells.
BRCA2 damage prevents the normal repair of DNA damage.

Medical opinion is that these women should have mastectomies or take preventative tamoxifen! Be aware that tamoxifen has been classed, itself, as a carcinogen by the WHO. Cancer Research UK have a 'Bodicea' test that can help determine the risk in your family.

Women in the highest risk categories need to take the highest care of themselves. General antioxidant boosters and cancer preventative measures should be employed. Prevention is the key.

High doses of vitamin C have been shown to be especially effective in the prevention of breast cancer *and* in extending life expectancy of those already diagnosed.

Vitamin D is now thought to be very important both in prevention and in trying to beat breast cancer (Royal Marsden). Take daily fish oil supplements.

Other considerations:

a) The timing of a breast cancer operation within a woman's monthly cycle appears crucial to survival rates. Three studies (Hrushesky *et al* 1989; Cooper *et al*, Guys 1999; Imperial Cancer Reseach Nov 1999) have led to this conclusion from the latter: "Women having breast tumours removed during the follicular phase of their cycle (ie. days 3–12 when their oestrogen is high) have a 10-year survival rate of only 45 per cent, compared to a 10-year survival rate of 75 per cent for when having surgery during the luteal phase (when progesterone is high). Natural progesterone has protective benefits, unlike synthetic progesterone which is a cause for concern.

b) A team of researchers at the University of North Carolina has ruled out Tamoxifen for prevention usage. It concluded that whilst there was a 6 to 8.3 per cent benefit, side effects were relevant to 90 per cent of women and were too great (**icon** – November 2004). At Dukes they have also shown it increases the risk of strokes.

c) Mastectomies – a team of Italian researchers at the Milan Cancer Centre analysed 1173 women between 1964 and 1980 concluding that mastectomies – with no other treatment – may actually cause spread and relapse. They suggested the simultaneous use of drugs that restricted tumour blood supply might help (**icon** – 2005 Issue 1).

• Skin cancers and melanoma

Only a minority of skin cancers are melanomas, but they are the most dangerous. Recent research suggests that the risk of spread (metastasis) is linked to the depth of the mole.

New research from the NCI in the USA shows that a woman lying in the sun whilst taking the contraceptive pill has twice the risk of an equivalent woman not on the pill.

Furthermore, another study on skin cancer showed that people who overcame their skin cancer had a greater risk than normal of developing a second, completely different, cancer later in life. All of these were oestrogen driven.

Conventional wisdom says keep out of the sun, stay off sunbeds, and that the sudden growth in this disease is due to the increase in exotic holidays in mid-winter and the over-exposure of white bodies to extreme sun. May be.

Clearly from the oestrogen findings, it is very likely that out skins are increasingly 'predisposed' to sunlight by our increased 'oestrogen pools'. This is worsened by the findings that some chemical ingredients like parabens, used in sunscreens and anti-perspirants and a known oestrogen mimic, is found in all breast cancer cells; whether or not it is causal in any way has yet to be determined.

As if to confirm this may not be a simple case of 'too much sun' the *Journal of the National Cancer Inst.* (2005; 99, 195–209) quotes research in New Mexico where people who had high sun exposure were *less* likely to develop melanoma. This was thought to be due to the protection vitamin D levels created.

It really is imperative to build an anti-oestrogen campaign for yourself. Excess sunshine is just too simplistic and misleading as a cause.

Birmingham University are pioneering a technique which boosts the immune system specifically against melanoma without the use of drugs (**icon** – November 2003) and similar 'melanoma vaccines' are being developed using the patient's own cells, in the John Wayne Clinic, California.

Research is under way in Melbourne where they have produced a vaccine to stop reoccurrence (**icon** – 2005 Issue 1).

Another reason for increased susceptibility can be genetic in about 10 per cent of cases (Leeds University).

• Colon cancer; bowel cancer; stomach cancer

There is a lot of mythology about colon cancer. For example the leading UK charity provides the following advice:

- Cut animal fats and red meat
- Cut alcohol consumption
- Eat more vegetables and fibre
- Cut caffeine consumption
- Watch your weight
- Increase fluid intake and watch your bowel movements!

However the research evidence is somewhat different to this. For example:

a) In the large scale Iowa study there was no link between vegetable and fruit consumption and reduced risk. But recent US research (**icon** – 2005 Issue 1) has shown that three helpings of vegetables per day (not including potatoes) reduces risk by 40 per cent. There is however a clear link between garlic consumption and reduced levels of colon cancer.

b) Japanese research in 2004 shows that increased salt levels increase risk. 12–15 grams of salt consumed per day more than doubles risk.

c) Both animal fats and alcohol increase the production of a carcinogenic bile acid. Consuming these two 'foods' literally causes you to poison yourself. Omega 3 and vitamin D cause suppression of this acid. (Fish oils – but not natural cod liver oil unless supplemented – provide both.)

d) Several research studies confirm that localised inflammation and the formation of polyps are precursors to colon/bowel cancer. Aspirin is known to reduce this, as will the anti-inflammatory properties of Aloe Vera. Garlic, ginger and omega 3 may also help.

e) Folic acid has been clearly shown to reduce colon and bowel cancer.

f) Finally, everybody over 50 (but particularly men) can be annually screened. Sigmoidoscopy seems to be the favoured and safe method.

Yeasts and microbes can play a significant part in colon and stomach cancer risk. One doctor I talked with told me that when he removed sections of diseased intestine they were often heavily infected with yeasts.

So plan to go on an annual yeast purge of Pau d'Arco, garlic, wormwood, cinnamon and caprylic acid. Take acidophilus regularly and avoid antibiotics, steroids and the like.

While colon cancer has tended to be the preserve of older men, a growing area of the disease is pregnant women. In 2001 Birmingham University found that colon cancer was linked to localised oestrogen.

Increasingly there are fears that stomach cancer is linked to *Helicobacter pylori*. The bacterium was historically kept in check by stomach acid levels, but the diets of the over 50's (typically mixing carbohydrate and protein) exacerbates the body's natural tendency to produce less acid as we age. Acidophilus also keeps *Helicobacter pylori* in check, as does 'Goldenseal'. Again steroids, statins, antibiotics and poor diets have reduced acidophilus levels in our bodies. You can be tested for *Helicobacter pylori* and it responds to drugs and bismuth.

Nitrosamines have been linked with stomach and colon cancers. Typically burnt food, for example, from barbecues, has been implicated. Smoked meats and fish, meats preserved with nitrites and pickled food have also been found 'guilty' in both Japanese and American research.

Finally, the Medical Research Council has found that abnormal glucose metabolism seems to be linked to colorectal cancer. Diabetics were found to have three times normal levels. So watch your sugar consumption and do not eat big, high carbohydrate meals.

• Ovarian cancer

Research shows that there are several possible causes of ovarian cancer.

- Synthetic oestrogen (from the pill and HRT). Long-term usage of HRT has been linked to 40 to 70 per cent increases in risk.
- The sexually transmitted bacterium Chlamydia has also been shown to cause ovarian cancer.
- Talc or talcum powder is something else that has been named as a possible factor in ovarian cancer (CPC, USA).

- Excess dairy has been linked to an increased risk of ovarian cancer.

Our website (www.iconmag.co.uk) covers ovarian cancer extensively. The UK's National Institute for Clinical Excellence (NICE) has just added PLDH as a second treatment drug to the previously approved topotecan.

Meanwhile look at the breast cancer section and cut your oestrogen levels. Go to a homeopath for a Vega check-up to determine if Chlamydia is involved. They will have nosodes to help eradicate it.

• Lung cancer

A study from the M.D. Anderson Cancer Center in Texas has shown that there is evidence that lung cancer runs in families. But then so does smoking.

Macmillan recently have shown evidence that early diagnosis helps survival rates significantly, and new treatments are being developed all the time, for example, Memorial Sloan-Kettering's Evlotinib trials which look very encouraging.

Again, lung cancer is extensively covered in our website.

Smoking causes increased risk of lung cancer. However, even with a lowered incidence of smoking in Britain, lung cancer rates are still growing!

Other causes are radon and diesel fumes. Indeed, smoking coupled with radon or diesel fumes has been shown to considerably amplify the risks.

A few lung cancers may be caused by X-rays or occur a number of years after radiotherapy on breast tissue.

In January 2004 research showed that formaldehyde plays a part in lung cancer. Exposure to formaldehyde may be in the work place, or as commonplace as breathing the fumes from nail cleaners and polishes!

Recent Austrian research has shown that volatile organic carbons and toxic chemicals emitted from typical household bleaches and cleaners collect at the crossroads in lungs at 400 times the levels previously expected. The scientists called on governments to ban certain chemicals from high street products.

Clearly to prevent lung cancer:

a) Avoid smoking.
b) Avoid smoke filled places and people who smoke.
c) Have your house checked for radon. Carpets worsen levels of dust in the air as do closed windows and doors.
d) Avoid living in cities or next to main roads.

Other general cancer preventative steps like taking antioxidants pale into insignificance behind the above factors.

Women have a greater risk of smoking-induced lung cancer than men because they have two X chromosomes whilst men have only one. This doubles factors, found in the airways, that link to levels of lung cancer.

You should be aware that there is research suggesting smokers, or workers exposed to asbestos, have an increased risk of lung cancer if supplementing with beta-carotene. Don't smoke, don't work with asbestos, do take beta-carotene!

• Brain tumours

Brain tumours will shortly become the number one cause of child death in America, ahead of car accidents and leukaemia.

The standard approach is surgery, radiotherapy and chemotherapy, although patients should be quite clear: Chemotherapy rarely works. Indeed an article in **icon** by Professor Geoffrey Pilkington (Portsmouth) said no drugs worked, and an article in *The Lancet*, February 2004, supported this.

So what positive things can we do?

Firstly it is important to realise that the brain is a very fatty tissue and fats dissolve and hold toxins and chemicals more readily. Households that use garden pesticides increase the brain tumour risk of their children; nail parlours in the USA have staff whose risk is eight times normal; ibuprofen, antibiotics and aspartame have all been questioned, etc, etc.

So start by clearing all the toxins out of your life.

Second, there is much work on mobile phones and EMFs showing increased risk. Clear these out of your life and sleep in an EMF-free room.

Certain foodstuffs nourish the brain, for example, choline and inositol (soy lecithin/B vitamins), fish oils/omega 3, echinacea, and should be considered (echinacea for no more than 8 weeks). Mistletoe therapy has shown results with brain tumours, in German studies, as has hydrazine sulphate in Russian research.

Charlotte Gerson talks about a 30 per cent 'cure rate' with people using the Gerson Therapy, and we know the Plaskett Therapy (via the Nutritional Cancer Therapy Trust) also claims good results. Obviously both aim to clear the body of toxins and in some cases could be very successful.

Professor Pilkington (see Q48) in liaison with Professor Wilkie (University College, London), is pioneering work with Clomipramine. Early studies seem to suggest that this can at least 'hold' brain tumours and there is some indication that this almost 50-year-old antidepressant drug can interfere selectively with brain cancer cells, making this definitely a route worth exploring. Omega 3 and lecithin seem to help its action.

Meanwhile, at Anderson, UCLA and Dukes in the USA, trials are studying Tarceva, a new type of drug that targets the growth factor involved in brain tumours.

The best advice, as with all cancers, is clean up your life, kick out all the dietary (brain tumours may well be oestrogen-mimic driven) and environmental toxins, and take good antioxidants, fish oils and soy lecithin supplements. Psychological causal factors should not be underestimated in brain tumours.

• Cancers of the blood, kidneys and liver

Whilst many solid tumours are hormonally, and largely oestrogen driven, cancers of the blood tend to be more 'toxin driven'.

The Journal of the National Cancer Institute (2003: 95) reported that factory workers exposed to formaldehyde have a much higher risk of leukaemia and particularly myeloid leukaemia. But formaldehyde, in many guises, is also found in a whole host of toiletry, cosmetic and household products.

Farmers seem to have a higher risk of multiple myeloma, due to their use of pesticides and herbicides in the fields.

Dark hair dyes have been repeatedly linked to some lymphomas and some kidney and bladder cancers (*International Journal of Cancer*, 15).

We have much more information on all of these on our website.

Child leukaemia is particularly responsive to chemotherapy, but at the other extreme, chemotherapy merely seems to give multiple myeloma patients about another year of life expectancy (although thalidomide is making a 'comeback' here as a form of treatment).

There is no doubt, in all these forms of cancer, that the patient must make every attempt to clean out their liver, detox their blood and body and boost their immune system. Michael Gearin-Tosh, the Oxford don, who has survived multiple myeloma for over ten years has immersed himself in the Gerson Therapy, and one can see why it would work. In these conditions the body needs a complete detox, not more toxins.

One slightly bizarre story is worth passing on. A nurse in the USA contracted leukaemia and was treated successfully with chemotherapy. A few years later her cancer returned, this time in her liver. Again, chemotherapy was suggested. Instead she consulted a nutritionist/homeopath who told her she had a bad yeast infection. A simple treatment with three anti-fungal drugs and her 'liver cancer' had gone.

The curious thing was that she worked in a child leukaemia ward. She managed to persuade the doctors to give the same anti-yeast drugs to the patients there and they witnessed a 25 per cent clear-up rate.

We know yeasts are a problem in the Western world, and can produce severe toxins in the body. All cancer patients are advised to check for their presence with a homeopath and eradicate them urgently.

Information is being gleaned all the time. For example, only recently have there been studies indicating the significant benefits on leukaemia and liver cancers of vitamin K. Researchers at the Mayo Clinic in June 2004 found that 'epigallocatechin-3-gallate in green tea seems to stop leukaemia in its tracks by interefering with crucial communication signals'. Four to ten cups per day were recommended!

Q48. Conventional cancer 'cures' – what's the alternative?

In the UK, the holy trinity of surgery, radiotherapy and chemo-therapy is the core of orthodox cancer treatment. But we are much, much more conservative than our European neighbours. And, remember, they have higher five-year survival rates. In Austria herbs are still used in treatments, in Germany in many top clinics the doctors are also qualified homeopaths and use Vega analytical machines. In Russia there has been much work done on energy and bio-resonance, with machines that can recharge your cell's and your body's energy. They have also worked on natural agents that can be used to selectively kill off cancer cells. China is also looking at 'peptides' from cell walls that are known to kill cancer cells *in vitro*. They have gone further and injected such peptides into the blood system of tumours, or directly into tumours. The FDA in the USA has picked up this work and it is known to be effective. When will it surface?

Meanwhile, top cancer centre, the MD Anderson Cancer Center in Texas, is publicly stating that all the exciting develop-ments in cancer treatment are in areas other than chemotherapy.

Let us look at a few realistic developments:

(1) Pancreatic enzymes

One branch of the alternative/complementary clinics has developed its beliefs around the pancreas.

In 1906 a Scottish anatomist and embryologist, **John Beard**, expounded theories about foetal cells and how, although they are rapidly dividing at first, this rate of division is switched to a more normal growth rate by a controlling mechanism provided by the pancreas.

Indeed he showed that an abundance of pancreatic enzymes occured in the foetus at the same time as these 'stem cells' were switched off. Yet the foetus had no need for these digestive pan-creatic enzymes, as all its food came from its mother.

All through our lives, such stem cells remain in our bodies and normally are 'switched' over to form eye cells, lung cells or muscle cells.

His hypothesis was simple. The 'stem cells' under the influence of oestrogen multiply rapidly as they do in the embryo. So what if cancer was simply stem cells collecting in one place, stimulated by oestrogen and dividing rapidly never to be differentiated with normal, slower growing cells that die? Equally maybe pancreatic enzymes could 'switch off' this process and convert the stem cells into normal healthy cells.

Maybe the theory is not so absurd. In Science 2004, *Professor Timothy Wang of Columbia University reported that genetic changes in stem cells prevented their differentiation into 'normal' cells. In 'breakthrough research that could change the whole thinking on how cancer forms', Wang's team looked into gastric (colon) cancer and concluded that first there was inflammation. Then stem cells from the bone marrow rushed to heal and deal with the problem. But they remained as stem cells and divided rapidly leading to cancer.*

Beard's work was developed further by **Dr William Kelley** in America.

Kelley took the theory and added another dimension. He believed everyone of us has their own personal metabolic code. His aim was to find this unique metabolism and stimulate it to switch off the stem cells.

Kelley theorised that the formation of cancer was clear. **Excess female hormones were responsibile for changing a stem cell into a trophoblast cell.** In simple English, this means that cancer is the growth of 'baby' tissue, but at the wrong time and in the wrong place. It progresses because of a lack of cancer digesting enzymes in the body and Kelley believed the pancreas, through its enzymes, was the primary cancer fighter in the body. So his solution was to get pancreatic enzymes to the cancer site and inhibit the growth, but control the rate of attack, or toxins would flood the body and cause problems elsewhere. This controlled attack needed to be linked to an individual's personal metabolism.

Kelley's treatment was divided into five parts:

1. **Nutritional therapy** – to break down the cancer cells; megavitamins, minerals, high dose vitamin C, bioflavenoids, coenzymes, raw almonds, amino acids and raw beef formula with pancreatic enzymes.

2. **Detoxification** – to cleanse the dead cells and toxins from the body; laxative purges, Epsom salts, fasts, lemon juice, coffee enemas (for anything from three weeks to 12 months)

3. **Diet** – to rebalance the body, the cellular metabolism and the immune system; at the outset he advocated a strict vegetarian diet, but modified this as he identified different individual types. In all he ended up with 10 different diet types and 95 variations. All diets forbade processed foods, pesticide residues, refined foods, peanuts, milk etc. They did allow almonds, low protein grains, nuts, organic raw fruits and vegetables.

4. **Neurological stimulation** – to allow free flow of body energy, especially to cancer site; for example, using osteopaths, chiropractors or physiotherapists. (A modern equivalent might be the use of a cranial osteopath to manipulate not just the skeletal structure but the free-flow of body energy.)

5. **Spiritual** – to lift the spirits, and call upon the universal good; Kelley urged patients to trust in God, to read The Bible and to pray.

Kelley monitored a patient's progress using his own Kelley Malignancy System. Over a 20 year period he reputedly treated 455 patients with 26 different cancers and claimed excellent results.

Even Ernst Krebs (of B-17 fame) followed this view of the pancreas.

Dr Nicholas Gonzalez is a New York immunologist who has a clinic with Dr Linda Isaacs, working on illnesses from cancer to multiple sclerosis.

They have based their cancer treatment on Kelley's work,

which they have refined and added to.

Gonzalez treatment dispenses with the neurological and spiritual elements. As with Kelley, Gonzalez believes cancer can be eliminated by the patient's own body, if the intestines, liver, kidneys, lungs and blood are all detoxified and the body's acid/alkaline pH and mineral and enzyme strengths are all in balance.

He uses his own system of hair analysis for monitoring progress.

Dr Gonzalez himself has been working on cancers since 1981. The results of his first clinical trial were published in June 1999. The clinic treats all cancers, although the current clinical trial is based on pancreatic cancer and results to date show that whilst all the control sample of patients on orthodox treatment have died, only one of Gonzalez's patients out of forty-nine on his diet therapy has succumbed. This is after almost five years, under the strictest test conditions.

The Gonzalez regime has just three basic units each modified for the particular individual being treated.

1. **Detoxification** – involves procedures such as coffee enemas (twice per day) to clean, purify and re-energise the liver. This in turn clears toxins out and improves the efficiency of the whole system.

2. **Diet** – individually designed diets using organic foods are used. Refined foods (sugar, flour, grains) are avoided, as are all processed and synthetic foods. Whilst some patients are on vegan diets using high levels of raw foods, others might be allowed two to three helpings of red meat.

3. **Supplements** – large doses of vitamins and minerals are used, including trace elements. Plus concentrates from glands and antioxidants and pancreatic enzymes, which whilst working as digestive aids, are also believed to represent the body's main cancer defence system.

In fact, Gonzalez believes that pancreatic enzymes actually liquefy tumours. It is not unusual for a patient to take 150–180 supplements along with 45 gms of pancreatic enzymes spread throughout the day.

He has also produced detailed studies of 50 patients, showing that all are alive 10 years later. His contact details are www.dr-gonzalez.com.

(2) Photodynamic therapy (PDT)

The earliest experiments with PDT took place in 1903, since when there have been almost 3000 published scientific papers on the subject.

The principle is simple. Find an agent which you can inject into the bloodstream of a patient; an agent that will target cancer cells not healthy cells. Then shine light on the agent and excite it enough to destroy the cell around it. Bingo!

Indeed work on PDT carried on until the 1930s then fell out of favour when this new fashion for chemotherapy took hold. However by the early 1970s more proponents were using it to treat patients and with notable success.

Obviously the choice of agent is critical as is the frequency of light that will activate it. Deeper tumours need red light, whereas surface tumours need only light at the ultraviolet end of the spectrum.

Branded agents have been established, for example Photophrin, and chemical agents are being developed all the time.

The downsides to date have been:

- The agents are not selective enough – they go into one healthy cell for every four or five cancer cells.
- They stay in the body too long – leaving the body exposed, since even sunlight can activate most of them
- They tend to focus only on a localised tumour, when as we have said, cancer is systemic and there may be other 'hot spots' around the body.

However, the Russians in particular are developing agents (shades of James Bond here!) based on algae and chlorophyll. The Gray Cancer Institute in Middlesex, working with cancer Research UK, has also been working with these natural plant extracts. Chlorophyll is structurally similar to haemoglobin but its centre is a magnesium atom rather than an iron atom. So it can travel in the bloodstream in a non-toxic way.

In Ireland Dr Bill Porter and Dr Tom Clearey, a pharmacologist, have developed a single chlorophyll-based agent and registered it under the name Photo Flora.

It has a number of unique properties and like all chlorophyll products produces oxygen when light is shone on it, and cancer cells hate oxygen.

The Photo Flora seems to attach to the cancer cells selectively, and the accidental incorporation into healthy cells falls to approximately one in forty-five cells.

The good news as well is that the new agent starts its work almost immediately it enters the bloodstream (you need only swallow supplements rather than be injected), takes far less time to reach the cancer cells, and is eliminated from the body more quickly than previous agents.

This one hundred year old idea is suddenly full of promise as new, natural agents are being developed and yet more sophisticated laser and infra red light systems are used. The Dove Clinic in England, who have experience of PDT, will be using this new agent and treatment which is called Cytoluminescent Therapy (CLT).

(3) Bioresonance

Your body is made up of billions of atoms each with electrons flying around them like planets around the sun. All such electrons exert forces on each other, attracting or repelling. You are indeed bionic man.

These electrical forces build up throughout the body and, just as there is a magnetic field around a wire which has a current through it, there is a magnetic field around your body. We discussed this earlier in Section III.

The Russians have photographed your magnetic field or aura, the Americans have shown how, in fact, it becomes ill first. Declines in the energy field around certain parts of the body or certain organs are inexorably linked to disease.

A number of scientists in America and Russia, for example, have also shown that a sick cell loses its electrical force, in the same way a battery might run out of charge. The power stations in every cell, if they become polluted, use less oxygen and produce less energy. They literally 'power down'.

When the cell loses its charge there is not enough energy to power certain genes, the most important of which – a gene called *p53* – is in the blue part of your DNA and acts to repair damage to the cell. A lack of charge means the cell cannot repair and defend itself.

Back in 1931, Dr Royal Rife developed a breakthrough microscope. Using this he claimed there was a virus at the heart of every cancer tumour.

He then identified a resonant frequency which, when he sent it into the tumour, excited the virus and caused its self-destruction. He then developed frequencies for all means of cancer viruses and microbes.

By the mid-1930s he brought his work to the world. However, until 1971 when he died, he was ridiculed, attacked and even witnessed his offices ransacked and burnt down such was the controversy he caused with the powers that be.

James Bare took his work forward in Canada and had his Rife-Bare machine approved by Health Canada (the equivalent of America's FDA), although he makes no claims for curing cancer. The original work by Rife featured 16 successful case studies.

Resonance machines, or zappers, are increasingly used to kill off yeasts and parasites. However, a lot of work is being done in Russia on killing cancer cells with such energetic frequencies, and this includes the idea of using them to recharge cancer cells back to their normal state.

Enter Dr David Walker. A Professor of Biophysics in the USA with minors in biochemistry and nutrition, Dr Walker himself developed colon cancer. After orthodox treatment failed he was told there was nothing more that could be done for him.

He then developed a three-pronged attack to cure himself.

- Nutrition – including glycoproteins, phytonutrients, antioxidants.
- Oxygenation of his system – including taking an enzyme, sodium micelle. (In the UK, you could instead try Zel-oxygen.)

- Re-energising his cells – using a self-designed resonance machine.

As a biophysicist he knew that a normal cell had around 70 microvolts charge, whilst a cancer cell just 15. At that low level the repair genes could not work, but the genes causing cell division thrived. So he set out to recharge his cells.

He cured himself and his fame grew. So he started helping other people. It wasn't long before the authorities took him and his extraordinary cancer treatment to court, but with 400 case histories and over 2500 testimonials, he defeated almost all the charges save two, that he had been prescribing treatments.

He is now 'over the border' in Mexico and his email is dlwalker@prodigy.net.mx

(4) Metabolic therapy

We talked about B-17 in Q17. Probably the lead exponent of this therapy is Dr Francisco Contreras, a Mexican, at his clinic The Oasis of Hope (www.oasisofhope.com).

His clinic uses the best of orthodox medicine combined with complementary therapies (for example, prayer, laughter and a modified Gerson nutritional therapy) plus alternative therapies such as laetrile.

The treatment is usually developed in conjunction with vitamin C megadoses, enzymes such as bromelain and papain and a total metabolic package. He feels that B-17 can work on all cancers save for brain tumours, sarcomas and liver cancers.

Metabolic therapy was a phrase coined by Dr Contreras Senior and really stands for a lot more than just B-17 treatment. There is no doubt that the Oasis of Hope, which is reviewed carefully by the medical authorities, has its successes and a full review is available on our website, www.iconmag.co.uk

(5) Vitamin C megadoses

Dr Patrick Kingsley works near Leicester in England. He treats a whole spectrum of patients, some of whom have cancer. These patients may or may not have had orthodox medical treatment first.

An open-minded gentleman, Dr Kingsley has no one treatment. He believes in identifying the cause of the cancer and what might be sustaining it and then treating that cancer with the appropriate mix of diet and therapy. He encourages positive thinking and historically has used a wide variety of treatments from B-17 to digestive enzymes.

One possible treatment, for example, is intravenous use of megadose vitamin C and hydrogen peroxide. The theory runs that the peroxide oxygen attacks the fastest growing cells in the body and cancer cells are killed by oxygen, whilst the vitamin C protects the normal cells from danger.

His diet recommends avoiding tea, coffee, milk and all dairy, wheat and yeasts, refined carbohydrates, sugars and junk food. He advises consumption of soya products, fresh organic fruits and vegetables (especially cruciferous e.g. broccoli, cabbage) and 10 gms of Ester-C per day (Ester-C is the non-acid version of vitamin C and supposedly kinder on the stomach) with large amounts of antioxidant vitamins plus 7–10 gms of echinacea. He also uses coffee enemas.

One report suggested he had a two-third success rate.

(6) Dendritic cell therapy

Dr Julian Kenyon at the Dove Clinic, Winchester also used B-17 therapy prior to June 2004 and a number of other therapies including vitamin C megadoses and Ukraine integrated with orthodox treatments. He currently works with PDT.

The Dove Clinic has also developed a new treatment based around the work of Professor Gus Dalgleish at St George's Hospital, London.

Professor Dalgleish has been looking at collecting a patient's own cancer cells in order to develop a specific vaccine. This vaccine then stimulates the patient's immune system to kick out the cancer.

The original problem is that often the cancer possesses the ability to hide from the immune system and protect itself. This requires that the immune system has to be refocused to recognise these abnormal cells.

Dr Kenyon collects compounds from the patient's own urine after treating the patient with megadose vitamin C, and then prepares the vaccines.

(7) Anti-neoplastons

A Polish doctor Burzynski, was fascinated by the fact that cancer patients lacked certain peptides normally found in the urine of normal healthy people. (Peptides are small chains of amino acids; over 30 the chains are called proteins.) He identified these peptides, which he called anti-neoplastons, and formed two 'packages' from the missing products.

All his early work concentrated on brain tumours, astrocytomas and glioblastomas, but recently he has developed 12 different packages each for various different cancers.

Early results showed a 50 per cent success rate for brain tumours, which if confirmed, would be a breakthrough.

At this point the FDA stepped in and ten years of court action took place. In the end he defeated all the charges and now continues with his work treating cancer patients, with his results monitored by the FDA. Hopefully soon we will have proper data with which to measure his success. His clinic is in Texas (www.burzynski.com).

Far more information and ideas from around the world are contained in our new book *Conventional Cancer 'Cures' – What's the Alternative?* published in January 2005. However, we pass these few examples on to you the reader so that you can realise that there is a wealth of opportunities and ideas being developed right now, some of which may be appropriate to you.

Hope springs eternal – for those with open minds!

SECTION VI

You really can beat
cancer

A summary

Introduction

If you want to beat cancer and you live in the West you need to be radical, disciplined and dedicate some serious time, effort and love to yourself. You must create your own micro-environment within a world that is increasingly full of dangers and attempt to reverse the surrounding trend of worsening odds, for yourself and those you love. You must start by reviewing your whole life.

Here are the five key principles:

Your diet

o *Get back to basics with simple fresh foods and base your diet around fruit, vegetables and whole brown rice*
o *Cut out the 'bad guys' (especially smoking, alcohol, sugar and caffeine) and introduce the good guys (see diet page)*
o *Supplement, detox and cleanse parasites and yeasts.*

Your lifestyle

o *Exercise daily; think slim*
o *Take up t'ai chi and/or yoga*
o *Go for three monthly body energy checks*
o *Cut the problems out of your life, or at least manage them better*
o *Reduce the risks of catching viruses.*

Your environment

o *Review all your household, cosmetic and toiletry products*
o *Avoid all radiation and magnetic fields*
o *Avoid all drugs whenever possible*
o *Avoid strong sunlight.*

Your mind

o *Learn to meditate*
o *List your strengths; develop your self-worth and self-esteem*
o *Take time for yourself*
o *Develop a plan for the future and a sense of purpose.*

Your soul

o *Think about your place in the Universe, now and in the future. Think about religion*
o *Practise acts of kindness, be friendly, helpful, look for strengths in others, use your own.*

Summary 1

How to beat cancer:
the 30 point checklist for everybody

1. Avoid fats and oils where possible, especially animal fats, and fats and oils in cooking. Use olive oil if you need to, but in moderation.
2. Do not smoke.
3. Reduce alcohol intake to two to three glasses of Cabernet Sauvignon per week.
4. Do not be overweight. Ideally be 5 per cent underweight for your height.
5. Eat nourishingly. Consume more carbohydrate and less animal protein. Consume more vegetables, fruits and rice, plus garlic and ginger. Think vegetables and fruit first. Have three meat-free days per week.
6. Ideally consume slightly less calories than you need per day. Eat six small meals rather than three big ones.
7. Eat raw, steamed, roasted but not microwaved, fried or barbecued food.
8. Juice fresh fruits and vegetables yourself
9. Try to avoid dairy, even small amounts; beware hidden dairy in cakes and biscuits, for example. Increase your consumption of pulses, including a little soya.
10. Don't drink fizzy soft drinks, especially low calorie ones
11. Avoid sugar, salt and caffeine. Drink green tea. Beware hidden salt and sugar in breakfast cereals or processed foods and remember mass produced juices are big sources of sugar.
12. Remove products which contain carcinogens from your everyday life.
13. Avoid electromagnetic radiation, near the house or in the bedroom. Beware mobile phones and radon.
14. Avoid all drugs where possible; avoid antibiotics
15. Be monogamous.
16. Women should avoid extra oestrogen e.g. the pill or HRT

17. Check regularly (once a year) for virus or parasite problems; keep yeasts at bay; take acidophilus.
18. Take cod liver oil every day.
19. Take supplements, especially the magnificent six. Have short periods during the year when you boost your herbal intake, especially astragalus, Essiac and echinacea, particularly if you've been unwell.
20. Drink filtered water from glass bottles.
21. Spend one hour a day looking after yourself.
22. Take some exercise daily. Try to exercise for seven hours a week. Do some resistance training.
23. Have a body energy service regularly, for example, every three months, with a cranial osteopath and/or an acupuncturist.
24. Love your lymph and move it daily with yoga exercises or some t'ai chi.
25. Calm yourself, free your brain, learn to relax, learn to meditate.
26. Learn about yourself, write a checklist of the things (including people) that limit you and avoid them. Don't put up with things that make you unhappy or depressed. Never feel guilty, subservient, desperate to please others or indebted. See friends, go to the gym, see a counsellor and/or doctor. Concentrate on the things that you enjoy and are your skills.
27. Establish your sense of purpose. What do you really want to be doing in three years or with the rest of your life? Write it down and stick it on the bathroom wall so you read it every morning. Remember. You can do it, or you can make excuses.
28. Discover your own spirituality. Think about how you interact with others; your body energy, inside and outside of you; think about how it interacts with the universe. Consider God and a religion. Practise acts of kindness, be helpful and understanding.
29. Fill your days with happiness and real value. Keep moving forward, don't live in the past.
30. Celebrate life.

Summary 2

Supplements:
the checklist for non-sufferers

Remember, nothing beats the real foods as they will always contain many more active ingredients. The following is a list of products with which to supplement your diet each day:

Beta-carotene	6–12 mgs (take during the day e.g. 3 x 4 mgs or 2 x 6 mgs)
Vitamin C	1 gm time-released (including rosehips/bioflavonoids)
Vitamin E	400 IU (286 mgs)
Zinc	15–25 mgs
Selenium	50–150 mcgs (max 200 mcgs)
CoQ10	30 mgs
Soya lecithin	3 gms max
Soya isoflavones	2 gms max
Garlic tablets	2–3 x 600 mgs tablets (equivalent to 500 gm of fresh clove)
Cod liver oil or fish oils	1,000 mgs

Doses given are for adults only. For children please consult your physician. People under 20 should not take CoQ10. Do not take large doses, over 5 gms, of vitamin C if you have been diagnosed with a primary or secondary brain tumour; it can cause asterocytosis in high doses.

Plus a good multivitamin and multimineral supplement (ideally colloidal) that contains B vitamins and folic acid (400 mcgs) plus traces of a wide range of minerals and amino acids.

Men can also take lycopene (10–20 mgs) and saw palmetto (400 mgs)

Consider eating apricot kernels (5–10 a day) and taking astragalus, echinacea and Essiac, especially if you've been unwell.

And if you don't eat much fruit, drink Noni juice and take aloe vera.

Summary 3

The action checklist for the cancer sufferer

NB This assumes a programme of surgery, then radiotherapy, then chemotherapy. See section IV for more details; you may also find that our simple hand-book *Cancer – Your First 15 Steps* helps you plan your personal programme in all its aspects.

Phase A   Diagnosis

1. Get a 'buddy'.
2. Develop a plan with your doctor and your 'buddy'. Try to work out what caused your cancer and what might be sustaining it.
3. Check everything you are told; get a second opinion, go on the internet. Demand answers.
4. Go for a virus, parasite and yeast check.
5. Cut out all possible carcinogens from your world immediately:

   - smoking, alcohol, caffeine, the pill, HRT
   - sugar, salt, preservatives, dried/smoked meats, crisps and snack foods
   - all dairy (including live yoghurt)
   - all refined and processed foods
   - all fried foods, all fats and oils, except olive oil
   - all red meats, farmed meats and farmed fish; go organic
   - your mobile phone, cordless phone, take the TV from the bedroom, don't sleep between lights, on or off
   - clear your house and garden of toxins

6. Start taking gentle exercise every day, if you've done none before. Go to a yoga class, learn to meditate. In 10 weeks going three times per week you'll be good enough!
7. Find a cranial osteopath, acupuncturist, homeopath and visualiser all of whom have experience dealing with cancer and ideally your sort.
8. Buy a three to ten day detox. Take daily, to help your liver

252

- 200 mgs milk-thistle (*Silybum marianum*)
- 3 gms soya lecithin
- Test your pH and alkalise your body via diet, or supplements like coral calcium and carctol.

9. Use the diet plan in the book and add in the following supplements:

– Fish oil	1,000 mgs per day
– Beta-carotene	2–3 x 6 mgs per day at intervals
– Vitamin C	1–3 x 1 gm per day at intervals
– Vitamin E	400–1,000 IU per day
– Zinc	1–3 x 15 mgs
– Selenium	200 mcgs
– Coenzyme Q10	30 mgs per day (especially if you are over 50)
– Lycopene	15–25 mgs

- 2 x 2 Garlic tablets per day
- A colloidal multivitamin, mineral and amino acid supplement (preferably containing no iron).

Doses given are for adults only. For children please consult your physician. People under 20 should not take CoQ10. Some supplements may conflict with some drugs.

10. Take 3 gms soya isoflavones per day.
11. Change to green tea, Essiac and drink at least 1.5 litres of water per day. Take astragalus and echinacea.
12. Consider taking Noni juice and apricot kernels. Use the list of alkaline producing foods. Eat garlic and ginger; take acidophilus.
13. Take linusit (2 tablespoons) with breakfast; or psyllium pills.

It is a lot to take but you need to boost your defences as quickly and as effectively as possible.

Phase B   Surgery

14. Keep with the plan above plus
    – buy vitamin E cream to reduce scars
    – think about talking with a homeopath to aid recovery

Phase C   Radiotherapy approaching

15. Detox three to five days.
16. Buy aloe vera gel to put on target area.
17. Look into supplements like MGN-3.

Phase D   During radiotherapy and after for four to six weeks

18. Go with someone to every session. Do not miss a session.
19. Take the supplements previously listed **especially** selenium, soya isoflavones and astragalus.
20. Keep taking your antioxidants and vitamin D. The latest research shows they improve results. Always tell your doctor.
21. The multivitamin and multimineral may now contain iron.
22. Eat lots of organic eggs and raw garlic. Take kelp or chlorella supplements and extra folic acid (in total about 800 mcgs – there were 400 mcgs in the multivitamin). All of this will help your hair stay in place and help protect your good DNA.
23. Increase water intake to 3 litres per day.
24. Keep up the yoga if possible; and especially the meditation and visualisation.

Phase E   After the radiotherapy has ceased to work

25. Talk to the doctor about your progress; get other opinions.
26. Get back to exercise and yoga. See the cranial osteopath, acupuncturist, healer and homeopath again, and get another programme sorted out.
27. Rebuild both your strength and your personal life.
28. Keep with the plan for diet and supplements in Phase A Definitely take:

    – Echinacea
    – Astralagus
    – Cat's claw

    If your cancer is hormonally driven look into natural progesterone cream or wild yam.

29. Keep any yeasts and parasites at bay.
30. Take some organic iron for seven days to boost your blood count.

Phase F   Chemotherapy

NB The run up to chemotherapy, the course and then the activity afterwards are more dependent upon the actual drug used, so you must consult your doctor.

31. Check any proposed drug on the internet. Get a second opinion
32. By and large repeat the radiotherapy plan.
33. Certainly look into MGN-3 and carctol as supporting agents for your immune system. Take vitamin K.

Phase G   Establishing your new life

34. Remember all those promises you made to yourself.......
    'When I get better, I'm going to ...?' Stick to your new life plan, your new diet, your new activities. Keep the bad things out of your life. New goals, new sense of purpose. Be happy with who you are, not who you think others want you to be
35. Celebrate life.

Don't eat	Do eat
Any farmed meat; red meat	Free range chickens, ducks, game
Any farmed fish, prawns, coastal fish	Deep sea caught fish
Any dried meats, cooked meats or sausages, smoked meats or fish	Have vegetarian days – two or three days a week
Any dairy, milk, cheese, margarine, yoghurts	All soya, tofu, tempeh, miso, soya sauce (Shoyu & Tamari)
Live yoghurt	Acidophilus
Ice cream	Sorbet
Dips	Hummous in olive oil
Fast food	The fish from fish & chips (if you have to)
Refined wheat, flour, sugar & salt; processed foods, chips, junk food	Oats, buckwheat, millet, organic brown rice (complete), fresh foods
Wheat, breakfast cereals, muesli	Home made cereal
Crisps, peanuts	Pumpkin/sunflower & sesame seeds, organic dried fruits
Chocolate, coffee, tea	Home made lemon & ginger & honey; Cassie tea, green tea with lemon grass
Cakes, biscuits, white bread	10 helpings of fruit and vegetables per day
E numbers	Garlic, chives, onions and leeks
Oranges, lemons, rhubarb, tomatoes (don't eat too many)	Bean sprouts, alfalfa, fennel, grilled tomatoes
Tap water in plastic bottles	Filtered boiled water. Glass bottled water
Barbecued or boiled or fried or microwaved food	Steam, roast, stew if you can't eat raw!
Gelatine	Agar-agar

A diet plan checklist

Why?
Farmed meat contains added hormones, antibiotics and pesticides from fields; cook well to destroy natural hormones.
Farmed fish (most prawns and salmon are farmed) again contains antibiotics and colorants. Coastal fish contain many toxins. Deep sea oily fish that has been caught is excellent (when eating out).
Dried meats and sausages again can contain antibiotics and added growth hormones, but also preservatives and nitrites.
Milk (even goat's milk) contains hormones, antibiotics and pesticides. IGF-1 from milk directly linked to cancers in prostate and breast. Soya contains active cancer blockers.
Dairy as above
Dairy as above
Chickpeas contain isoflavones which block tumours.
Fast food is often cooked in hydrogenated vegetable oil which spreads free radicals, hits the immune system and makes bad eicosanoids.
Processed food, sugar & salt weaken the immune system. Should eat organic whole brown rice each day; eat fresh foods, nourishing foods and build your body energy.
Sprinkle linseeds (Linusit), millet bran, pumpkin seeds, sunflower & sesame seeds over oats for breakfast. Use Soya milk and honey to sweeten.
Hydrogenated oils, salt, preservatives & colouring replaced by organic natural sources of vitamin E & isoflavones. Crisps, chips, cereals, biscuits contain acrylamides.
Chocolate, coffee, tea are no-go areas. Green tea with lemon grass is a real antioxidant mixture, as is Cassie tea or: pour hot water onto slices of fresh lemon and ginger with a little honey.
Cakes, biscuits contain fats & milk. White bread is refined and full of salt, sugar & preservatives. Beware brown bread – look for *wholegrain, wholemeal*. Try lemon grass, Brussels sprouts, cabbage, broccoli, kale, apricots, peaches, pineapples and papaya (red & yellow fruits and veg). Salads of avocados, red and yellow peppers, watercress, herbs, carrots.
Do not overcook or you will lose the anti-cancer agents allicin, selenium, germanium, L-cystine.
These fruits are good in moderation but very acid. Try juicing watercress & fennel or green apples (organic without wax or preservatives). Alfalfa is highly nutritious, as are bean sprouts.
Aviod parasites and nasty minerals. Avoid toxins from plastic bottles; filter your own water.
Eating raw vegetables before meal gives you 40 per cent more vitamins; fried gives you bad oils; overboiling takes away vitamins; barbecued makes carcinogens (nitrosamines).
Swap the animal fat out of your cooking.

THE POSTSCRIPT

Catherine's 'survival'

The 31 August 2001 was Catherine's 23rd birthday. The evening before, she was given her first 'all clear'. One presumes that this is what is termed 'remission', but they used no such couched jargon, simply the words all clear. The MRI scan showed the scar tissue from her operation, a large number of dead cancer cells but none that was living or growing.

Three months later another scan still failed to find any cancer cells, as did another in May 2002. One eminent surgeon following the case described this as 'a miracle'. Apparently he had been told things were pretty hopeless and that she had less than six months to live back in May 2001. No one said anything like this to us at the time, but whatever we thought or feared was anyway lost under a mountain of determination, teamwork and effort.

Perhaps I should provide a little more information and detail.

When Catherine was told she needed surgery, we urgently put her on 1 gm of time-released vitamin C a day, 1,000 mgs of cod liver oil, 1,000 IU of vitamin E and 30 mgs zinc. This little cocktail and Mr Kitchen's excellent work with the knife were responsible for almost negligible scarring despite a cut from the centre of her crown to below her ear just in front of the hairline.

But there was more. Fearing the worst from day one, two weeks before anyone mentioned the dreaded 'C' word, we added to the above, 15 mgs beta-carotene, 200 mcgs of selenium, plus Neway's Maximol, a quality colloidal multivitamin with minerals and amino acids, 15 mgs lycopene and 30 mgs Coenzyme Q10 simply to boost her immune system on a daily basis.

By the time the worst was confirmed we had received some serious supplies of supplements and also had a theory for how her illness had come about.

No-one in the medical profession seemed bothered about what had caused Catherine's brain tumour. Catherine ate no fruit, she used a mobile phone to the tune of £150 plus per month, was on the pill and drank to excess like most other female students. I must admit I was shocked when I found out she also smoked up

259

to 25 cigarettes a day. She talked a good exercise class but I doubt she participated too often, and she also had a fairly typical cancer sufferer's psychological profile. She liked to please everyone else, put herself bottom of the list, did things for peer group approval and often felt guilty about letting people down when she clearly hadn't. Catherine certainly had the odds stacked against her.

There was however another factor that worried me. In her first 18 months of university (about three years previously) she had had tonsillitis frequently. She had had this illness all her life, but only once a year. At university she was having it every twelve weeks. The doctors were prescribing the usual amoxycillin and she would take Ibuprofen.

Then I read an article about yeasts and how, if you take lots of antibiotics, the good bacteria in your stomach were killed, allowing the yeasts to come out to play. So two years ago she started taking caprylic acid, oregano, garlic and Pau d'Arco, with a ban on wheat (previously her favourite foods were pasta, bread and pizza) for the summer. The result was that she recovered and had 10 months tonsillitis-free. When it did recur she went to a cranial osteopath who said that my solution was pretty well right but gave her a longer list of ingredients to avoid, and moved her body energy around as it was concentrated in her overactive stomach area, with none around her head and neck. The result. No more tonsillitis.

However I now believe that greater effects were already taking place in her body.

Yeasts are notorious weakeners of the immune system, which is one reason the tonsillitis continually reappeared. They drain the body of all vitamins, particularly B vitamins. Catherine's lifestyle of tobacco, alcohol, stress, lack of sleep and the pill would have seen off any vitamin B that did actually make it past the yeasts.

But B complex vitamins include three components essential to DNA and the brain. Folic acid is essential for the accurate replication of DNA in dividing cells. Choline and inositol are rare in that they can pass through the blood/brain barrier and they are known to nourish the brain cells.

Worse, in the American book 'Brain Fitness' the two authors

Dr Klatz and Dr Goldman describe antibiotics and anti-inflammatories as two of their six 'brain poisons' and antibiotics are known to prevent proper absorption of folic acid. All this was building up a picture of why she may have had this failure in her left frontal lobe. (I should add that if mobile phones were linked to brain tumours, experts believe they would more likely appear at the side of the head.) Another possible cause, Aspartame, is being studied in research in the UK right now but I had told the children my fears about Aspartame four years before and they had ceased drinking diet drinks.

Rather like Dr Jane Plant in her book, my view was, 'If we can work out a likely cause, we can also work out what is sustaining the cancer and act upon that.'

My theory led me to write a diet for Catherine, a modified and more general version of which appears in this book. My principles for Catherine were:

- kill off the yeasts and any parasites
- return a good supply of Vitamin B especially to the brain
- remove all antibiotics from the diet
- cut all the toxins out of her life
- give her an alkaline body
- rebuild her immune system and strengthen her for the inevitable radiotherapy.

The anti-yeast programme meant removing all dairy, wheat and sugar from the diet, stopping all alcohol, eating no mushrooms, marrow's, courgettes, melons, cucumber, fruit juices and fruits (easy for Catherine) and taking caprylic acid, Pau d'Arco, garlic, Echinacea and acidophilus.

For a multivitamin and mineral supplement she took four units of Neway's Maximol, colloidal liquid per day. This had several benefits. Catherine was taking enough pills already and it was a liquid; the list of contents was amazingly comprehensive covering amino acids as well as minerals and vitamins; it contained fulvate/fulvic acid which is the naturally occurring active ingredient in plant roots that enables minerals to pass more easily from the soil into the plant; and finally it is a colloidal suspension of a type known to be easily absorbed.

I did however add a B complex every two days for its folic acid content and gave her soya lecithin (for inositol and choline) and soya isoflavones.

As antioxidants we gave her 400 IU of vitamin E, 1 gm of vitamin C (time release) and 2 x 6 mgs beta-carotene. She was also taking 200 mcgs selenium and coenzyme Q10 30mgs and 25 mgs lycopene.

She took 1,000 mgs of cod liver oil every two days to try and reduce and replace her 'bad fats' content with omega 3 and enhance her vitamin A levels to fight the cancer.

Her diet was changed to reflect all this with much more fresh garlic, olive oil, salads and fish. We bought her lemongrass and galanga, green teas and Essiac, replaced all the milk with soya and she cut out caffeine and sugar.

She was given a bowl containing pumpkin seeds and sunflower seeds to munch instead of crisps. And chocolate, tea, coffee and dairy were banned. Her consumption of water rose markedly and she took Neway's Noni juice as I was very worried about her lack of fruit consumption and the likelihood of her body being on the acid side of the desired pH line.

As I was concerned about the possibility of parasites linked to cancer, she also took an anti-parasite product, Neway's purge.

Yes, she was taking a lot of supplements but we were in an urgent and corrective situation.

Her radiotherapy lasted six weeks, she went to every session and someone always went with her for mental and moral support.

By now she was tired and had lost her hair. Some days her depression was so evident you could have weighed it.

During the last two weeks of radiotherapy we talked a lot. We stayed together in London and went to the tennis at Wimbledon, saw 'Mamma Mia', and 'Chicago' and we did fun things. We talked through an idea to produce a regular magazine for doctors and patients alike on all the latest developments in cancer; be it about clinical trials on drugs in Boston or successful case histories on visualisation techniques at Bristol.

I had been busy trying to track down a supplier of B-17 but had run up against the FDA bans. But a friend who had spare apricot kernels – her sister in America was sending them for their mother's cancer (with great success I must add) – provided a pack of those. This, if nothing else, saved my mother from eating apricots and banging the stones open with a hammer in the back garden every day! From about week four of the radiotherapy Catherine started to eat 30 kernels a day and take bromelain and papain supplements (Oh, that she would eat pineapple or papaya!).

When the radiotherapy finished, we went to my house in France for a month with her sisters and brother and a selection of girl friends, and had some fun and fresh air. We used the time to refocus Catherine on her future happiness, lifestyle and sense of purpose. I couldn't stop Catherine drinking Rosé, but on top of her normal supplements we reintroduced beta-carotene (2 x 6 mgs) but this time in the form of Neway's Cascading Revenol which has beta-carotene and a mix of other antioxidants, plus astralagus, cat's claw, wild yam, lycopene and organic iron (the latter just for one week) all to rebuild her immune system and her blood count as fast as possible. I just used to hand her different pills at different times of the day so I'm not even sure she knew what she was taking. Except that it was a lot.

I had finally managed to get hold of some B-17, having chased round the internet. Catherine took 6 x 500 mgs tablets a day, plus 6 tablets of Megazyme, a mixture of bromelain, papain, pancreatic enzymes and other helpful ingredients. She did, however, use the B-17 pills as an excuse to give up the apricot kernels, which were too bitter for her liking.

Interestingly when she saw her oncologist for a routine update meeting, he blamed her heartburn on 'the B-17 turning to hydrogen cyanide in her stomach'. It doesn't.

Catherine also refocused her lifestyle. The smoking, the pill and most of the dairy consumption went. She took to the gym very regularly and attended three yoga classes a week. Her weight (she was never particularly overweight) has tumbled from the steroid induced size of Autumn 2001. She is back at work full-time and has had a full, successful and productive 2002.

Who knows what worked in this cocktail of radiotherapy, fun and supplements? Do I care? Well, yes actually I do. I genuinely wish I could say it was a combination of these two or three things so that others could really benefit from our knowledge. All I can

263

say is, 'Somewhere in this mix, a combination of factors seemed to deliver a result and ... so far, so good'.

I saw Catherine just after the New Year festivities in 2003, a year and a half after her diagnosed 'time limit', and with four all clears behind her. But, she was eating a hamburger, and her boyfriend was chain smoking next to her. "How was Christmas?" I asked. "Wonderful, I got pissed every night" came the reply. I suppose at 24 you think you are immortal. Catherine had even ceased taking the supplements.

Shortly afterwards she lost her speech for 30 seconds. The tumour was back. It was so hard to keep Catherine on some sort of programme. The euphoria of four 'all clears' had quite literally gone to her head.

During the early days of her illness, we had come across Clomipramine. Professor Pilkington was preparing trials on this 45-year-old anti-depressant, which he felt might work against the unique power stations of brain cancer cells. I spoke at the National Brain Tumour conference and one of the other speakers did a whole presentation on the possibilities for this relatively mild drug.

However Catherine's oncologist sat down with her and said he had a combination of three drugs with which he was achieving a 70 per cent success. Although I advised against it, Catherine took the drugs and was so ill she couldn't even take a second round. Her immune system was shot to pieces.

Catherine then decided to take Clomipramine and took a number of supplements from parasite killers to wormwood (a blood test showed she had bad yeasts again) and MGN-3, cat's claw and even some organic iron and astragalus to get her white cells back up. (The hospital had been providing her with phials so she could inject herself to re-stimulate her white cells, but to little avail.) A little Noni, Maximol and Revenol were the basics in the programme and she went back to the gym and her healer.

But by March 2004, one year later, the tumour had grown again. Another operation. The interesting thing was that the tumour had grown but not spread. Catherine celebrated three years 'survival' in Ireland, where she had a course of photody-

namic therapy. But whilst we look at a seemingly never ending list of possible treatments around the world three conclusions are inescapable.

Firstly she is too slack with her supplements, whilst tubs of ice cream have found their way back into the diet. The thought of ever doing a coffee enema fills her with horror, and she publically states that she will do anything, AS LONG AS SHE CAN CONTINUE WITH HER LIFESTYLE! That is young people for you!!! My friends continually tell me that 'you're never a prophet in your own land' and they are right!

Secondly, in her first year she fought the tumour with a pretty good immune system. Recent blood tests confirm she now has no white natural killer (NK) cells. I believe this is the product of the chemotherapy, which in her case was totally useless. Now she is fighting the enemy within, using a catapult where once there were machine guns.

Finally, glioblastomas are bad news. Very bad news.

Sadly, Catherine passed away on October 22nd 2004. Her oncologist had originally predicted she would live six months – one summer – he has not known anyone live for longer than 18 months with a grade 4 glioblastoma.

Catherine survived three and a half years living a full and happy life. We miss her greatly.

Let everybody reading this book take the positive lessons from her story. A life, a full life, seven times longer than expertly predicted tells its own story. And there is every chance that you could do even better, if you are prepared to make the commitment and stick at it. We have learned so very much through all this. I hope you have too.

And Next?

I am convinced that across the hundreds of books written and the wealth of information on the internet, the solutions for cancer are already known; but some heads will have to be banged together to encourage a more genuine belief in this by the people officially in charge of our country's health. The medical profession has no exclusive mandate on curing cancer but sadly they are almost exclusively the focus of funding from the Government, drug companies and sponsors. It is hard to see how one oncologist could understand the full benefits of meditation or how a sense of purpose filters down from the brain to alter the biochemistry of a prostate cell. It is simply too big a subject for any one person to become a complete expert in.

At some point the status quo must change to provide genuine through the line teamwork that brings all the possible solutions together into a managed package for sufferers. Shouldn't every hospital cancer unit offer 'complementary help'? Shouldn't every hospital try to give you a personal manager who can help you get the best out of all the known treatments, be they radiotherapy or visualisation, vitamin supplementation, or analysis of possible causes?

Laurens Van der Post began a campaign in 1982 aimed at persuading the medical establishment to form closer ties with complementary practitioners. In 1998 the NHS approved £18.4m to renovate the Royal London Homeopathic Hospital, its 'principal complementary medicine provider' and in 2001 there were reports of the Prince of Wales backing Dr Mosaref Ali to form his integrated hospital. I am pleased to note Macmillan's 2002 directory of 300 complementary services in the UK, of which approximately one third are attached to hospitals and hospices. These are but small steps in the right direction.

My personal aim is to launch a 'centre of excellence' in the UK for information on all forms of cancer therapy so that people can make more informed decisions and build their own 'personal prescriptions' that give them the best chances of success with their cancer. But the first real step that needs to be taken is a decision to be more open-minded to the possibility that some of these alternatives might have merit. And, like America, we then need an independent body to both fund and properly trial all complementary and alternative therapies.

Next, we need doctors to understand that the first step in any treatment programme should be the revitalisation of the patient's

immune system. Their natural defence against cancer. Only there-
after should the orthodox medicine start.

Finally the Government should pledge a large sum of money for
the next 50 years to finance an independent body to review, and
have the power to tackle, prevention issues. This should be inde-
pendent of the medical profession, the Government, the health
service and the drugs companies. The body should be allowed to
have real control and to properly use the law and even change it
when, for example, it sees toxins being used in everyday products
or produced by factories, it wants hard facts on the long term
effect of pesticides or GM foods, or it feels there are health consid-
erations on electromagnetic fields which should over-rule current
planning approvals on pylons and transmitters by local authorities
made only on aesthetic grounds. It would be a massive undertak-
ing and one that might take time to bring results even if the will
were there, but it is absolutely essential to the future health of the
nation. The recent Macmillan review concluded that by 2025 the
number of cancer cases each year would double, and this would
almost certainly bankrupt the NHS. To tackle prevention head-on
seems a win-win situation to me.

But the truth is to really achieve results we have to cut the crap
and clear out the people who have vested (and often secret)
interests from the overall decision-making process.

We need a body that is the people's champion and doesn't have
the slightest hint of any relationship with any one with any inter-
est, other than the genuine desire to reduce the levels of cancer
contracted in the future.

Having spent the last three years immersed in this vast and
complex world of cancer, I am convinced cancer can be beaten
and the truth is we probably know enough already to do it. But
the increasingly myopic, 'orthodox' route we are taking now
simply cannot be right for either us or our children. We need
open-mindedness, a new order, a step change. And I hope you
agree that, in this book, there is more than enough evidence to
support my view that the fight against cancer is a "winnable' war.

Chris Woollams
March 2005

APPENDICES

APPENDIX I

Acid Residue Producers - a fuller list

FRUITS

Bananas
Grapefruit
Oranges
Plums
Prunes

VEGETABLES

Asparagus tips
Brussel sprouts
Chick peas
Dried beans
Lentils
Peanuts
Rhubarb
Tomatoes

ALL DAIRY

ALL FLESH FOODS

Meats, fish, shellfish, scallops, crab,
All processed and salted meats, smoked fish

CEREALS AND NUTS

All packet nuts, crisps and snacks
All refined flour including noodles, spaghetti, buckwheat
Barley
Cornflakes and most processed breakfast cereals
Doughnuts
Dumplings
Macaroni
Oatmeal
Pies, pastries and bread
Refined rice

OTHER

All alcohol
Chocolate, cocoa
Coffee, tea
Fizzy drinks
Eggs
Lack of sleep
Negative emotions
Preservatives, jams etc.
Products in vinegar
Salt and condiments; MSG
Sauces
Stress
Sugar
Sweets
Tobacco
Vinegar

Alkaline Residue Products - a fuller list

FRESH FRUITS

Apple	Lemons
Apricot	Lychees
Avocado	Mangoes
Blackberries	Melon
Blackcurrants	Olives
Cherries	Papaya
Cranberries	Peach
Currants, raisins	Pear
Dates	Raspberries
Figs	Redcurrants
Grapes	

OTHER

Alfalfa	Honey
Agar-Agar	Millet
Fresh cracked nuts	Noni juice
Fresh ginger	Olive oil, corn oil
Fresh juices (own preparation)	Seeds
Herb teas, green tea	Soya products

VEGETABLES

Aubergines	Kale
Beetroot	Kelp
Broccoli	Lettuce
Cabbage	Mushrooms
Carrots, parsnips	Parsnips
Cauliflower	Peppers
Celery	Potatoes
Chard	Radishes
Chicory	Sorrel
Chives	Soya beans
Cucumber	Spinach
Dandelion	Squash
Dill	Swede
Endive	Turnips
Fresh green beans	Watercress
Garlic	

APPENDIX II

Useful Contacts

Telephone

a) Cancer Helplines – Specific

Bladder Cancer	0207 831 9831
Brain Tumours (S D R T)	01252 627 426
Breast Cancer Care Helpline	0808 800 6000
Colon Cancer Helpline	0207 381 4711
International Myeloma Foundation	0800 980 3332
Kidney Cancer UK	0247 647 4993
Leukaemia Research Fund	0207 269 9068
Lung Cancer (Roy Castle Foundation)	0871 220 5426
Ovarian Cancer UK	0207 380 9589
Pancreatic Cancer	0121 449 0667
Prostate Cancer Helpline	0845 300 8383

b) Cancer Helplines – Complementary & Integrated

Breast Cancer Haven	0207 384 0000
Bristol Cancer Centre Helpline	0117 980 9500
Gerson UK	01372 817 652
The Dove Clinic	01962 718 000
The Hale Clinic	0870 167 6667
The Nutritional Cancer Therapy Trust	01636 612 707
The Institute for Complementary Medicines	0207 237 5165

c) Cancer Helplines – General

Cancer BACUP Helpline	0808 800 1234
Cancer Research UK	0207 061 8355
Cancerlink Helpline	0808 808 0000
Cancer Resource Centre	0207 924 3924
Macmillan Cancer Relief	0808 808 2020
Marie Curie Cancer Care	0800 716 146
The Patients Association	0208 423 8999 OR 08456 084 455

British Acupuncture Council 0208 735 0400
The Association and Register of Colonic
  Hydrotherapists 0870 241 6567
The Society of Homeopaths 0845 450 6611
The British Federation of Massage Practitioners 0177 288 1063
The British Assn of Nutritional Therapists 0870 606 1284
Institute for Optimum Nutrition 0208 877 9993
National Radiological Protection Board 0800 614 529
The Sutherland Society (Cranial Osteopathy) 0122 5869 100

Websites and Doctors

1. General Sites

Cancer Guide
www.cancerguide.org
This site gives you info on how to find what you want and get the best possible treatments.

Cancer Bacup
www.cancerbacup.org.uk
The UK's leading information service. Very professional, regularly updated with tailor made service, publications, nurse and links to other sites. Top notch with over 100 local centres throughout the UK. Good for rare cancers.

Cancer Research UK
www.cancerresearchuk.org
Largest cancer charity in Europe with a site to match. Latest news, links to specific sites. 'Everything you need to know about cancer' (now, where have we heard that before!)

National Cancer Institute
www.nci.nih.gov
A bit formal, US site covering all cancer types with treatment information, news on latest development projects and trials. Massive.

American Cancer Society
www.cancer.org
The definitive US site; news, information, and latest developments. Easy to use.

Royal Marsden Hospital
www.royalmarsden.org
Brilliant site from UK's top cancer unit. Find out about everything jargon-free. Good information booklets, latest news.

Memorial Sloan-Kettering
www.mskcc.org
New York gold standard cancer treatment centre with information to match. Very clinical.

2. Carers, Self Help and Home Support

Macmillan Cancer relief
www.macmillan.org.uk
Support for people with cancer and their families. Aim to provide best support, treatment and care. Access to 2000 nurses for community and home help.

Marie Curie
www.mariecurie.org.uk
Care for thousands of people in their own homes and at hospices throughout the UK.

3. Integrated and Complementary

M D Anderson Cancer Center, Texas
www.mdanderson.org
Leading US Cancer Centre. Also has state of the art Integrated Cancer Treatment Centre.

The Bristol Cancer Help Centre
www.bristolcancerhelp.org
'We practice, teach, research and develop the holistic approach as an integral part of cancer care'. The professionals.

Breast Cancer Haven
www.thehaventrust.org.uk
Breast cancer site with emphasis on complementary therapies, counselling, and support services.

The Dove Clinic for Integrated Medicine
www.doveclinic.com
Screening, complementary treatment including dendritic cell therapy and light therapy plus counselling in London and Winchester.

Gerson Therapy
www.gerson.org
American site offering advice on the treatment, with newsletter and books

Nutritional Cancer Therapy Trust
www.defeatingcancer.co.uk
UK site covering nutritional therapy and based on Dr Plaskett's revisions to, and updating of, Gerson.

Dr Gonzalez
www.dr.gonzalez.com
The alternative cancer centre in New York that will officially prove diet therapy can beat orthodox treatments.

Dr Walker
Tel: +52 622 226 0390
Energy resonance, diet and ozygen therapy tailored to the individual.

Burzynski Clinic
www.burzynski.com
The use of peptides to make up for shortfall in cancer patients.

Dr Patrick Kingsley
Tel: 01530 223 622
Integrated approach to causes and possible cures.

Dr Contreras
www.oasisofhope.com
The number one integrated clinic in the world. Everything from chemotherapy to metabolic therapy.

4. Specific

Brain
www.sdrt.co.uk
UK independent site, helpful with good research list.

Breast – Breast care
www.breastcancercare.org.uk
Free publications and booklets. Refer you to phone line. Good link to-

The Lavender Trust
www.lavendertrustfund.org.uk
Breast cancer site aimed at the problems faced by younger women, with great details on benefits and state financial assistance.

Colon
www.coloncancer.org.uk
Excellent and frequently updated site, offering news research and advice.

Leukaemia
www.leukaemia.org
(USA) Information for new patients, research, news and support systems.

Lung cancer
www.roycastle.org.
The Roy Castle Lung Cancer Foundation is the only charity in the world dedicated to lung cancer; support groups, dedicated nurses, research, even quit smoking programs.

Melanoma
www.cancer.org.au
Australians know more about melanoma than anyone.

Myeloma
www.myeloma.org
Truly international site, with information on new treatments and own magazine; style, a bit formal.

Oral

www.dentalhealth.org

Information on oral cancers and treatment available in the UK from the British Dental Health Foundation.

Ovarian

www.ovacome.org.uk

UK wide support group for all those concerned with ovarian cancer.

www.ovarian.org

(US site). Information, help and clinical trials.

Pancreatic

www.pancan.org

(US site). Help for patients and their families.

Prostate

www.prostate-cancer.org.uk

Bright lively site with information, help, and chat lines and message boards. Order leaflets and info packs on-line. Excellent.

5. Clinical Trials

European Clinical Trials

www.EORTC.be

Monitors clinical trials, the development of new drugs, and other innovative approaches to improve the standard of cancer treatment in Europe.

Worldwide

www.nci.nih.gov

American top site for clinical trials.

APPENDIX III
A selection of books you might read

Your Body's Energy	Emma Mitchell
Chakra Healing	Liz Simpson
Ayurvedic Home Remedies	Vasant Lad
Natural Detox	Marie Farquharson
Fit for Life	Marilyn Diamond
Instant Calm	Paul Wilson
The Road Less Travelled	M Scott Peck
Take Time for Your Life	Cheryl Richardson
Vibrational Medicine	Dr Richard Gerber
Food, Your Miracle Medicine	Jean Carter
Ageless Body, Timeless Mind	Deepak Chopra
Your Life in Your Hands	Professor Jane Plant
The Cancer Prevention Diet	Dr Rosy Daniel
Stopping the Clock	Dr Ronald Klatz and Dr Robert Goldman
The Vitamin Bible	Earl Mindell
Foods That Fight Pain	Dr Neal Barnard
Hands of Light	Barbara Ann Brennan
The Safe Shopper's Bible	David Steinman and Samuel Epstein
A Cancer Battle Plan Sourcebook	Dave Frahm
Natural Compounds in Cancer Therapy	John Boik
Living Proof: A Medical Mutiny	Michael Gearin-Tosh
Eat Right For Your Type	Dr Peter J D'Adamo
Oestrogen: The Killer in Our Midst	Chris Woollams
Cancer – Your First 15 Steps	Chris Woollams
The Tree of Life: The Anti-Cancer Diet	Chris Woollams
Conventional Cancer Cures – What's The Alternative?	Chris Woollams

APPENDIX IV

Liver Cleanse/Gallstone Flush

Ingredients:
$1/2$ cup extra virgin olive oil
1 very big grapefruit (providing $3/4$ cup of juice)
4 tablespoons of Epsom Salts
3 cup of water
Ornithine tablets.

Preparation:
Set aside three days.

Day 1:
Eat a no-fat breakfast; and lunch.
Eat and drink nothing after 2.00 pm.
Mix the Epsom Salts in the water (easier if water is warm), then cool.

6.00 pm	Drink a quarter of this liquid.
8.00 pm	Drink a further quarter of the liquid
10.00 pm	Mix the olive oil and pulp-free grapefruit juice and shake vigorously.
	Drink the liquid through a straw before 10.15 pm.
	Take four Ornithine tablets to help you sleep.
	Retire immediately and massage your stomach.
	Focus your mind on your liver and imagine the toxins leaving it, along with the stones.
	Sleep.

Day 2:
Upon waking and not before 7.00 am take the third quarter of the Epsom salts mix. Two hours later take the last quarter.

Expect diarrhoea for two days; don't eat before lunch time on day two and keep food to salads and fruit, plus baked potatoes for days two and three.

You may need to repeat this treatment after a few weeks. 2000–3000 small stones may be passed.

Please note – This recipe is derived from William Kelley's cancer treatment. It has thousands of testimonials, none reports pain, only success; but nobody at Health Issues has any first hand experience of it. We are merely **told** it works!

To order more copies of this book

Tel: 44(0)1280 815166

Fax: 44(0)1280 824655

E-mail: enquiries@iconmag.co.uk

icon magazine
(integrated cancer and oncology news)

For the latest information,
breakthroughs and news on
cancer prevention and cure,
see icon magazine

For a free trial copy ring:
Tel: 44(0)1280 821211

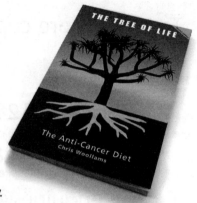

OESTROGEN
THE KILLER IN OUR MIDST
by
Chris Woollams

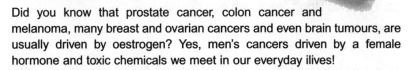

"This book is amazing – it told me things I had no idea about"   Dr J.H. (Salisbury)

Did you know that prostate cancer, colon cancer and melanoma, many breast and ovarian cancers and even brain tumours, are usually driven by oestrogen? Yes, men's cancers driven by a female hormone and toxic chemicals we meet in our everyday ilives!

Some specialists believe 90 per cent of solid cancers are hormonally driven and 90 per cent of these we prove are driven by oestrogen. And this is true for both men and women,

Most usually this is a **breast** cancer but it can be **prostate** cancer, **colon** cancer, **melanoma**, a **brain tumour** or **ovarian** cancer.

Without a doubt the 'driver' is invariably an oestrogen.

Chris says: *"This book is a very important book for anyone with a solid tumour. It is meant to be very easy and quick to read, but to clearly cover the facts and suggest what action you might take to amplify your orthodox treatment. Things most doctors simply do not tell you. It will also save me a lot of time, hormonally driven cancer is so common I have often had the same conversation five times in just a few hours!"*

Oestrogen: The Killer in Our Midst is a self-help book for all those wishing to beat or avoid hormonally responsive cancer.

"It's easy to read and with a checklist of action points. It pulls all the information together in a usable way."   E.T. (Hertfordshire)

"I think it's invaluable for anyone, male or female. It covers everything from cutting oestrogen excesses out of your life to the use of natural progesterone. I didn't realise that there is so much you can do."   P. F. (Limerick, Eire)

Tel: 44(0)1280 815166

Fax: 44(0)1280 824655

E-mail: enquiries@iconmag.co.uk

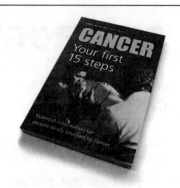

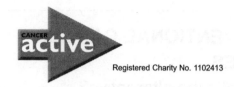

CANCERactive is a new charity with three important points of difference.

• First, it brings you the WHOLE TRUTH ON CANCER TREATMENTS: all the up-to-date facts about every researched therapy that might be of help to you. From surgery to supplements; from radiotherapy to exercise; from chemotherapy to photodynamic therapy. We don't show bias, we just lay out the facts so you can choose.

• Second, it is dedicated to helping people build an INTEGRATED treatment programme, to maximise their chances of survival. Books, a magazine (**icon**) and an easy-to-follow website are all packed with information and our own research is planned.

• Third, it aims to take the PREVENTION message where it matters, into schools and to parents.

BECOME AN ACTIVIST – JOIN THE FORCE

For just 50 pence per week you can join the FORCE, and receive **icon** posted to your home, a monthly e-newsletter, discounts on health products and a whole lot more.

 "Everything you need to know to help you beat cancer."

Now no one need die of ignorance

Tel: 44(0)1280 821211
Fax: 44(0)1280 824655
E-mail: enquiries@canceractive.com